Nightingale's Legacy

Nightingale's Legacy

The Evolution of American Nurse Leaders

Sue Johnson, PhD, RN, NE-BC

American Nurses Association

Silver Spring Maryland • 2016

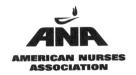

AMERICAN NURSES
ASSOCIATION

American Nurses Association
8515 Georgia Avenue, Suite 400
Silver Spring, MD 20910-3492
1-800-274-4ANA
http://www.Nursingworld.org

The American Nurses Association (ANA) is the only full-service professional organization representing the interests of the nation's 3.4 million registered nurses through its constituent/state nurses associations and its organizational affiliates. The ANA advances the nursing profession by fostering high standards of nursing practice, promoting the rights of nurses in the workplace, projecting a positive and realistic view of nursing, and by lobbying the Congress and regulatory agencies on healthcare issues affecting nurses and the public.

Cataloging-in-Publication Data on file with the Library of Congress

ISBN-13: 978-1-55810-627-7   SAN: 851-3481   1.0K   1/2016

First printing: January 2016

Contents

Introduction   vii

1. Linda Richards: A Nightingale Nurse 1

2. Clara Barton: America's Florence Nightingale 7

3. Mary Eliza Mahoney: America's First Trained African American Nurse .. 15

4. Lillian Wald: Urban Crusader 19

5. Mary Adelaide Nutting: Nurse Scholar 27

6. Lavinia Lloyd Dock: Activist and Historian 33

7. Annie Warburton Goodrich: Pacifist and Patriot 37

8. Isabel Hampton Robb: Nursing Visionary 43

9. Mary Breckinridge: Pioneer in Maternal–Child Advocacy 49

10. Margaret Sanger: Family Planning Activist 63

11. Estelle Massey Riddle Osborne: Administrator and Change Agent 77

12. Mabel Keaton Staupers: Organizer and Negotiator 85

13. Mary Elizabeth Carnegie: Educator and Editor 95

14.   Susie Walking Bear Yellowtail: Grandmother of
      American Indian Nurses 105

15.   Madeleine Leininger: Founder of Transcultural Nursing 111

16.   Virginia Henderson: First Lady of Nursing 119

17.   Luther Christman: Nursing Visionary 125

18.   Richard Carmona: Always a Nurse 135

19.   Eugene Sawicki: Priest and Nurse 145

20.   Peter Buerhaus: Nursing Workforce Scholar 153

      Epilogue   159

      Afterword: Nightingale Legacy Leaders and Nurse Leadership
      Competencies   163

      References   167

      Index   175

Introduction

Life is made of the past, present and the
future. We're shaped by our past, and we're
shaping our future with our present.

—Ibrahim Emile

Florence Nightingale's legacy has been advanced by American nurse leaders—some famous, some relatively unknown—over the past 160 years and counting.[1] Each of these leaders contributed significantly to both the nursing profession and health care, using varied approaches to advocate for individuals, communities, racial and ethnic groups, and—most importantly—for patients. Their impact continues to influence the practice of today's nurse leaders even though many of today's leaders are unaware of the significance of these 20 American nurse leaders. It is imperative that our current and future nurse leaders understand these accomplishments and leverage them in the future for the nursing profession to thrive throughout the 21st century.

1.   The year 1855 was in many ways the beginning of Florence Nightingale's legacy. It saw the culmination of her work in the Crimean War, which realized immediate benefits for the wounded and sick of that war as well as long-reaching changes for improved public health and health care, and what would one day become the profession of nursing. In November of that year, the Nightingale Fund was established in recognition for her work. By the end of the decade, she had used a substantial part of that fund to found a training school for nurses in London. This was the only recognition of her services that Nightingale would approve (Selanders, n.d; see also Dossey, 2000, pp. 156–168).

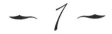

Linda Richards

A Nightingale Nurse

(July 27, 1841–April 16, 1930)

Linda's Story

Linda Richards grew up in an era when American nurses were totally untrained and unprepared to care for the sick patients in their charge. The majority of these nurses were more concerned with themselves than providing patient care or alleviating pain. They administered unlabeled medications without any knowledge of proper dosage or the effects on patients in large hospital wards. This carelessness and absence of concern resulted in a lack of respect from physicians (Richards, 1911).

There were a few bright spots in this grim period in health care and nursing. One was Linda Richards, who was recognized as a "born nurse" from her teens (Richards, 1911, p. 3). This term depicted a dedicated, kind, positive, cheerful woman who loved nursing and gained experience from older women and family doctors. The born nurse was always on call and devoted herself to the needs of ill individuals.

Richards gained some experience caring for sick neighbors, but wanted to enter a hospital and really learn how to be a nurse. The problem was that there were no nursing schools in the mid-1860s. She started her career as an assistant nurse at Boston City Hospital. Richards's position was similar to today's housekeeping aides, and she found that most of her colleagues were not observant and lacked common sense when providing care (Richards, 1911). She left after three months to seek a place that would teach her the skills she needed to truly care for patients.

Richards went to the Hospital for Women and Children in Boston and was the first person to enroll in the first class of five nurses in the first American training school there. Life was hard for these students in the one-year course. Richards and the others worked from 0530 to 2100 taking care of six patients each. They stayed in little rooms between the wards and frequently were called at night for patient care. Every second week, they were off duty from 1400 to 1700 one afternoon. Except for that small break, they had no evenings or Sundays off, no hours for study or recreation, and no pay for the first three months. Richards's first formal exposure to nursing education included limited instruction in medical, surgical, and OB with lectures by visiting physicians. Female interns showed the nurses how to do temperatures, pulses, and respirations (TPRs) and assigned duties. There were no textbooks and no entrance or final exams and, as the first applicant, Richards was the first to graduate (Richards, 1911).

After graduation, Richards became the night superintendent of Bellevue Hospital Training School. All orders and reports were verbal and she created the first written case notes there, a beginning point for today's written documentation and bedside charting. She also began class instruction for nurses in training and after a year was asked to be the superintendent of the training school at Massachusetts General Hospital (MGH). Richards gained the support of the physician superintendent and they arranged for physicians to give lectures to the nurses in training. The program was a success, but Richards still wasn't satisfied with her own knowledge and skills (Richards, 1911).

In 1877, the Massachusetts General Hospital (MGH) school and trustees arranged for Richards to spend time in England to gain experience at hospital training schools. In May, Richards met with a small lady in black with black kid gloves and deep blue eyes—Florence Nightingale (Richards, 1911). Nightingale had arranged funding for the St. Thomas' Hospital Training School from the Nightingale Fund established for her during the Crimean War (Cook, 1913b). Now, she and the Matron there arranged for Richards to spend a week in each of the eight wards and to attend numerous operations. After four days at St. Thomas, Richards was invited to Nightingale's home and impressed her with her desire to learn training school leadership. Nightingale recommended that Richards spend time at King's College Hospital and the Royal Infirmary of Edinburgh and wrote the following letter of recommendation to the Matron at the Royal Infirmary: "A Miss Richards, a Boston lady, training matron to the Massachusetts General Hospital, has in a very spirited manner come to us for training to herself. She would have taken the ordinary year's training with us, but her authorities would not hear of it, and we admitted her as a visitor. I have seen her, and have seldom seen anyone who struck me as so admirable. I think we have as much to learn from her as she from us." (Richards, 1911, p. xxiv–ix)

With this high introduction, Richards spent a month at King's College Hospital doing patient care and at the Royal Infirmary, where she saw her first typhus case and learned about Joseph Lister's aseptic treatment of wounds. Richards also impressed the superintendent of the Royal Infirmary, who told her "I find you a superintendent of a training school, and one who is well trained and seems to understand her work well" (Richards, 1911, p. 48).

After these experiences, Richards visited Nightingale at Lea Hurst and discussed the comparison between American and English/Scottish training schools. Nightingale offered sage advice and Richards went to Paris for a month to visit hospitals there before returning home. As she headed home, she received a letter from Nightingale with the following challenge: "May you outstrip us, that we may outstrip you" (Richards, 1911, p. 53).

In late 1877, Richards accepted the challenge to help develop a training school for nurses at Boston City Hospital. She was supported by the physician superintendent, but not by the 10 house officers and their 3 assistants. Many of the nurses found the two-year course too difficult and left. Six nurses completed the rigorous program, which included nurses taking vital signs, charting, and preparing dressings. By the end of the first year, even Richards's opponents acknowledged that patients received better care from the training school nurses (Richards, 1911).

In 1885, the American Board of Missions advertised for an experienced nurse to develop a training school in Japan. Richards accepted the position and went to Japan alone to begin her new mission. She studied the language and culture and, with the help of an interpreter and female missionary, began classes for 5 Japanese nurses. This experiment blossomed and by September 1887, there was a junior class of 13 women, and several other training schools were established by the Japanese in other towns. Richards's nurses became superintendents of these training schools. In June 1888, an important moment in Japanese history occurred when 4 Japanese graduate nurses received their diplomas. The fifth original student couldn't complete the course for health reasons. The school and its graduates were respected and the Japanese maintained Richards's high standards, the high quality of nursing care, and benefits to patients (Richards, 1911).

Richards also lifted these Japanese women from total subservience to educated professionals. When a Japanese woman visited Boston City Hospital after Richards's return, she remarked upon Richards's dedication: "You left this beautiful place to go to live in Japan, where everything is so small and poor. The difference between you and Moses is that he went to his own people and you went to strangers" (Richards, 1911, p. 102).

Richards's nursing career after her return from Japan included multiple leadership positions to organize training schools in both general hospitals and psychiatric hospitals in the East and Midwest. Her philosophy that nurses must continue to gain knowledge and work as individuals to rapidly grow "the art of caring for the sick" (Richards, 1911, p. 116) became the mantra for future nurse leaders.

Richards herself summed up her nursing career with the following statement: "I have found life full of interest in an earnest endeavor to do faithfully my small part in the great movement which has resulted in establishing the profession of the trained nurse in America" (Richards, 1911, p. 117).

Implications for Nurse Leaders Today and in the Future
Individual Recordkeeping System for Patients

Nurse leaders are aware of the importance of documentation in their organizations. Comprehensive patient records are essential for provision of quality care, communication about patient needs and concerns, and reimbursement for services. U.S. organizations are moving rapidly toward electronic medical records (EMRs) that surpass Richards's handwritten chart, but the principle remains the same—a comprehensive chart available to all providers for the patient's benefit. As the movement toward EMRs gains acceptance, nurse leaders must consider benefit–cost analysis and return on investment for selected systems. Converting to an integrated system with an EMR, central data repository, and clinical decision support is necessary to ensure interoperability that will result in healthcare savings and safety benefits (Hillestad et al., 2005). Nurse leaders must be involved in decision-making on EMR systems and computerized physician order entry (CPOE) to ensure that orders are legible and accurate.

We have come a long way since Linda Richards's peers administered unlabeled medication based only on verbal orders. We have an opportunity to reduce medication error rates and the incidence of adverse drug reactions as we move from paper documentation to health information technology. Nurse leaders also must consider other potential benefits from disease prevention interventions and chronic disease management (Hillestad et al., 2005). Electronic triggers can alert physicians and other health providers by recommending preventative services (e.g., cancer screening, vaccinations) and coordinating workflows for higher-risk patients (e.g., communication between multiple specialists and patients). Nurse leaders realize the costs inherent in integrated EMR systems, but must be cognizant of the benefits to patients from reduced hospitalizations and an emphasis on prevention. Linda Richards's creation of an individual record keeping system for patients has evolved to the movement toward EMRs. Now, nurse leaders must ensure that these interoperable EMR systems produce the efficiency and safety results and savings that they should (Hillestad et al., 2005).

Global Collaboration

Today's nurse leaders understand the importance of formal education for nurses. In Linda Richards's era, little to no formal education was available. Now, we have multiple avenues to attain a nursing degree and the Institute of Medicine's recommendation that nurses should practice fully based on their training and education as full partners with physicians and other healthcare professionals echoes Linda Richards's and Florence Nightingale's emphasis on the importance of trained nurses (Institute of Medicine, 2011). Nurse leaders have an obligation to encourage and support nurses in attaining additional formal education to benefit the profession and particularly the patients.

Linda Richards's success in founding and supervising the first training school for nurses in Japan is relevant to today's nurse leaders. Nursing and patient care are global and nurse leaders have opportunities to share information with colleagues in distant lands. Some American hospitals are also interacting with sister hospitals overseas to address professional issues. One example is MGH, where Linda Richards was superintendent of the training school for nurses in the 1800s. The scale of MGH's Professional Practice Environment model has been used to develop a Chinese version that enabled Taiwanese nurses to evaluate healthcare system changes and their practice environments (Ives Erickson, Jones, & Ditomassi, 2013). Although regional issues may differ, there are common priorities that nurse leaders can address globally to impact practice settings and meet current and future challenges in nursing and health care internationally (Ives Erickson et al., 2013). This is an opportunity for nurse leaders to achieve global success as Linda Richards did in Japan. She pointed the way and it is the responsibility of nurse leaders to continue international collaboration for the benefit of nurses and patients worldwide.

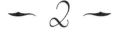

Clara Barton
America's Florence Nightingale

(December 25, 1821–April 12, 1912)

Clara's Story

Clara Barton came to nursing in a roundabout way. The youngest of five children, she was separated from her closest sibling by about a dozen years. It was a boisterous household where it was difficult for Barton to establish a place for herself. A shy, timid child, she excelled in school, but felt inferior to her older brothers and sisters and compensated by engaging in activities with male cousins. She became a proficient horsewoman and even attempted ice-skating, an activity not allowed for women (Barton, 1907).

When Barton was 12, her brother, David, was hurt in a barn-raising accident. For the next two years, she devoted herself to nursing David back to health. This set the pattern for her life—a need for achievement, true compassion for the weak and disadvantaged, and dedication to philanthropy and a cause (Brown-Pryor, 1987). After David's recovery, she had to find a new purpose for herself. She and a neighbor girl nursed several families during a smallpox epidemic and Barton was warmly remembered for her efforts by members of those families (Brown-Pryor, 1987).

She still struggled with feelings of insecurity and began to identify her worth by being of service to others. Although well-educated among women of her era, Barton always believed that her education was inadequate. In spite of that, she became a teacher who was widely sought for her ability to engage students in learning. She was able to gain the respect and love of students who were too rowdy for other teachers. However, teaching was not satisfying to Barton as a career, although it was one of few choices for single women. When Barton and her brother, Stephen, advocated for a district school for millworkers' children in 1845, she was unable to deliver her written speech at a town meeting because she was a woman. This inequality continued when she established two successful schools, only to be replaced by a man in 1853. This rejection reinforced her belief in her own worth: "I shall never do a man's work for less than a man's pay" (Brown-Pryor, 1987, p. 23).

Unsure of her future, Barton moved to Washington in 1854 and found a job as a temporary clerk in the Patent Office. At first, she received a salary that was comparable to her male counterparts. However, when the commissioner of patents resigned, matters took a turn for the worse. The new commissioner gave the women in the Patent Office no work and Barton drew no salary for three months. She enlisted the support of her congressman and was able to pick up work at the office and be paid based on the amount completed. The former commissioner returned and Barton was returned to her former salary and position although the men working there resented her. The situation was exacerbated when she discovered and reported some of her male colleagues for illegally selling patent privileges. When the office of commissioner changed hands again, Barton was dismissed in August 1857 (Brown-Pryor, 1987).

For the next two years, Barton studied at a local academy, lived off her savings, and battled depression. She remained unsure of her future and her desire to help others was largely unfulfilled. Barton was relieved when she was recalled to the Patent Office in December 1860. This time she accepted the role of a temporary copyist at a lower salary and cultivated a friendship with Henry Wilson, the Senator from Massachusetts. With his support, she was confident that her job was now secure (Brown-Pryor, 1987).

Soon, Barton would become an active participant in a nationwide conflict—the American Civil War. In 1861, she began her work with the following statement: "I may be compelled to face danger, but never fear it and while our soldiers can stand and fight, I can stand and feed and nurse them "(Brown-Pryor, 1987, p. 80). For the remainder of the war, Clara Barton became famous for her battlefield visits and care for wounded and dying soldiers. She worked frequently without rest in terrible conditions and bought (or begged for) and delivered relief supplies that weren't supplied by Army quartermasters. Barton cleaned, cooked, and assisted with surgeries, and her presence boosted the morale of stricken soldiers (Brown-Pryor, 1987).

After the war, Barton worked for free to identify missing soldiers and finally was dismissed from the Patent Office, where she had been absent most of the war. She began to lecture about her war experiences and was well received by audiences. She also met Elizabeth Cady Stanton and Susan B. Anthony in 1867 and began a long relationship with them to promote women's rights. While they were focusing on suffrage, Barton began to champion rights for African Americans. In 1868, Barton's health at age 48 was suffering and her doctor recommended she go to Europe for rest. After trips to Scotland and England to stay with friends, Barton went briefly to Paris and Geneva in 1870, where she met for the first time with representatives of the International Convention of Geneva (Red Cross). It was the first time she had heard of this organization and she was impressed that they had warehouses filled with contributions from all of Europe to be used by whichever side needed them in wartime. They also had trained nurses: Barton met with the Grand Duchess Louise, the daughter of Kaiser Wilhelm, who encouraged women to participate in disaster relief and promoted the establishment of several nursing schools. She and Barton became friends, a friendship that would last both their lives. Barton became somewhat involved in relief work in Strasbourg, but found little government support in Paris for her efforts. Kaiser Wilhelm awarded her the Iron Cross of Germany, making her the first and only woman to receive this honor. Barton became ill and returned to London where she stayed a few blocks from Florence Nightingale, who declined to meet her. They exchanged a few notes and never communicated again (Brown-Pryor, 1987).

On her arrival home in 1873, Barton was honored in New York City and spent time in New England and Washington, where she became ill with bronchitis and was hospitalized. She spent time in a sanatorium in Dansville, New York, in 1874 for nervous exhaustion and emerged stronger and healthier two years later. Barton needed a new humanitarian challenge, at

56 years of age. She thought of forming an American Red Cross, and asked permission from the International body. The International Committee appointed her as their Washington representative and Barton began to develop a Red Cross for peacetime disaster relief as well as wartime relief efforts (Brown-Pryor, 1987).

The first branch of the American Red Cross started with 22 charter members on May 12, 1881. For the next 20 years, Clara Barton and a select group of supporters fought for official recognition through incorporation of the Red Cross and adoption of the Treaty of Geneva by the U.S. government. Both of these were essential to give the organization legal standing and government support. The United States had an isolationist approach to foreign entanglements at that time and the bureaucracy considered any agreement with a foreign nation a threat to America's autonomy. Barton lobbied Congress to adopt the Treaty of Geneva and her solo efforts resulted in ratification on March 16, 1882. This was a singular achievement for humanitarianism (Brown-Pryor, 1987).

Barton wanted a congressional charter and working funds appropriated from the government, but neither was forthcoming. She used her own funds to keep the organization afloat and, largely due to her efforts, the International Committee recognized the American Red Cross on June 9, 1882. Congress continued to see the Red Cross as a private organization and other rival organizations (e.g., the Blue Anchor, the White Cross) fought to assume this role in disaster relief. Each of these organizations eventually dissolved and the Red Cross responded at various levels to numerous national and international disasters for the next 20 years under Barton's presidency. She often went herself to distribute supplies and provide support. While she was warmly welcomed, the national organization was dependent on her to function. Even an able administrator would have had difficulty obtaining supplies, field staff, and financial resources as well as maintaining accurate records for this fledgling organization, and Barton found herself unable to deal with the administrative details or delegate. A powerful movement began within the Red Cross to reorganize and establish a sound financial foundation. Barton resisted as long as she could, but finally resigned on May 14, 1904 (Brown-Pryor, 1987).

She was still popular with the Grand Army of the Republic's veterans and feminist groups and remained active in their meetings. She lived simply and devoted her income from speaking engagements to funding the

National First Aid Association until the American Red Cross absorbed it in 1908. Clara Barton was dedicated to humanitarian causes and disaster relief when it was difficult for a woman to excel in these fields. The "Angel of the Battlefield" (Brown-Pryor, 1987, p. 99) would go down in history as a dedicated philanthropist and the founder of the American Red Cross (Brown-Pryor, 1987).

The parallels between Clara Barton—the "Angel of the Battlefield" (Brown-Pryor, 1987, p. 99)—and Florence Nightingale in the Crimea are striking. Both provided supplies from their own funds for wounded soldiers. Both engaged in relief work in hospitals and on the battlefield and worked tirelessly to nurse the wounded. The soldiers they nursed worshiped both of them. Both faced opposition from physicians and military leaders who didn't want women in hospitals. Both dealt with untrained personnel: Nightingale with orderlies (Cook, 1913a) and Barton with ambulance workers (Brown-Pryor, 1987). Both gained legendary status for their courage and dedication during their time spent in war zones (Cook, 1913a; Brown-Pryor, 1987). Both also were frequently ill throughout their lives and had dominant personalities that did not appreciate dissent (Cook, 1913a, 1913b; Brown-Pryor, 1987).

However, there were distinct differences between Barton and Nightingale. Florence Nightingale was raised in a wealthy British family and was financially secure throughout her lifetime. She was revered by wealthy, elite members of the ruling class (including the Royal Family) from her 30s until her death on August 13, 1910 (Cook, 1913b). Clara Barton frequently struggled to provide for herself as well as demonstrate philanthropy to others. Where Nightingale felt family love and support, Barton frequently was uncomfortable with her family and often felt lonely and isolated. She had few influential friends in the United States and little personal funds during her life. Barton struggled to prove her value in a country where women were not empowered and had difficulty delegating the advancement of her work to others (Brown-Pryor, 1987).

She summed up her life in the following sentence: "I have lived my life, well and ill, always less well than I wanted it to be, but it is, *as* it is, and as it has been; so *small* a thing to have had so much said about it" (Brown-Pryor, 1987, pp. ix–x).

Implications for Nurse Leaders Today and in the Future
The Importance of Delegation

Clara Barton was a gifted humanitarian and philanthropist who believed that only she could accomplish her work. She preferred to labor alone and surrounded herself with people who did as she directed them. This approach worked for a short time, but proved to be a major drawback in the development of the American Red Cross (Brown-Pryor, 1987). Today's nurse leaders also face situations daily that require delegation to succeed. It is imperative that nurse leaders clearly appreciate what delegation means to ensure correct and competent performance of delegated tasks and responsibilities as they decide what to delegate and to whom. This process begins by understanding the definition of delegation as a "transfer of responsibility for the performance of an activity from one individual to another, with the delegator retaining accountability for the outcome" (Wacker Guido, 2015, p. 76). Using this definition, responsibility for performing a task or action is transferred, but the delegator remains accountable for the results.

Nurse leaders realize that they cannot do everything alone, as Clara Barton tried to do, and must depend on others to achieve desired effects and success. They must clearly understand the impact of their personal leadership style, education, and confidence level in their ability to delegate to the correct individual(s). Delegation provides an opportunity to enhance communication effectiveness, develop positive working relationships, and increase trust. It requires experience and confidence that must grow with practice. An integral aspect of leadership is developing others to succeed. When the nurse leader communicates and delegates appropriately, the benefits to the patients, the delegatee, the unit, the facility, and the leader are remarkable (Wacker Guido, 2015).

Advocacy for Disaster Relief

Clara Barton's role in disaster relief, both in the Civil War and for many years after, is legendary. She positively changed numerous lives and established a foundation for philanthropy for disaster victims that continues today (Brown-Pryor, 1987). At some point in their career, each nurse leader will be confronted with a natural or manmade disaster. Healthcare facilities play a major role in preparation, response, and evaluation and follow-up when such disasters occur. Nurse leaders are responsible for emergency planning, staff awareness and preparation for their assigned roles, and resource allocation and training to implement timely intervention (American Nurses Association [ANA], 2015, p. 82). Organization leadership, including nurse leaders, at all levels must be knowledgeable about the organization's emergency plans, including division of responsibility, authority, and accountability. Review of emergency plans, surge capacity, emergency communications, and staff assignment or reassignment must occur on a regular basis accompanied by external and internal disaster drills. These approaches will facilitate prompt and competent response when an actual disaster does occur. The public expects healthcare organizations to address these major community threats capably (ANA, 2015b). The Standards of Professional Nursing Practice are applicable in disaster situations to guide nurse leaders in planning, providing, and evaluating disaster relief. These standards enable nurse leaders to collect and review applicable data, identify concerns or trends, identify expected outcomes, plan appropriate interventions, implement emergency plans, coordinate activities with other leaders and staff, educate healthcare team members, consult with safety experts, and evaluate outcomes to improve future responses (ANA, 2015b, pp. 4–5). The Standards of Professional Performance guide nurse leaders in preparing for disasters and disaster relief by assuring professional competence "related to ethics, culturally congruent practice, communication, collaboration, leadership, education, evidence-based practice and research, quality of practice, professional practice evaluation, resource utilization, and environmental health"(ANA, 2015b, p. 5).

— 3 —

Mary Eliza Mahoney

America's First Trained African American Nurse

(May 7, 1845–January 4, 1926)

Mary's Story

Mary Eliza Mahoney has the distinction of being the first African American trained nurse in the United States. She was the eldest of three children, whose parents migrated to New England from North Carolina as free African Americans. Mahoney was interested in nursing from an early age, but only one African American student was accepted yearly according to the charter of the New England Hospital for Women and Children (Hine, 1989). Mahoney had to earn her way to acceptance in this early training school. Starting at 18, she worked as an untrained practical nurse at this hospital in Roxbury. She also supplemented her meager income by working as a cook, janitor, and washerwoman (Campbell, 2012).

In 1878, Mahoney's efforts paid off and she was enrolled in the nursing program at the New England Hospital for Women and Children at age 33 (Campbell, 2012). The nursing program used students as unpaid workers and Mahoney was responsible for six patients during 16-hour days on the wards. In her limited time off, she was required to attend long lectures and study throughout the 16-month course. Students were always fatigued and many failed to complete the entire course. In her class, Mahoney was 1 of only 4 graduates from a class of 42. She proudly received her nursing certification on August 1, 1879, and became the first African American woman to attain her nursing license (Campbell, 2012).

Since hospitals did not hire staff nurses at that time, Mahoney registered with the Nurses Directory and did private duty nursing throughout the east coast for about 30 years. Her expertise was widely sought and she became a role model for other African American women who aspired to careers in nursing (Campbell, 2012; Davis, 1999). Mahoney advocated for racial equality in the nursing profession as well as women's equality and suffrage (Darraj, 2005; Davis, 1999). She was proud to cast her first vote in an election at age 76 (Carnegie, 1991).

Mahoney was an early supporter of a professional nursing association for women of color: the National Association of Colored Graduate Nurses (NACGN) that was founded in 1908 to improve working conditions for African American nurses (Campbell, 2012). The fledging organization's first national convention was held in Boston in 1909 and Mary Mahoney addressed the attendees with hopefulness for the future of African American graduate nurses. Mahoney "emerged as an ideal emblem of the aspirations and potential achievements of African-American nurses" (Darraj, 2005, p. 75).

Mahoney's life revolved around her patients, her church, and her limited private time to read. Her patients adored her and a New England Hospital staff member and colleague said "I used to hear her praises sung everywhere around Boston and suburbs" (Darraj, 2005, p. 55).

Mahoney was a proponent of equality and advancement for African American nurses, but her most important role was as a professional. Most of her nursing work was for white families. Early in her career, she was expected to perform domestic tasks as well as nursing duties. As her career progressed, Mahoney began to draw a line between the two roles. Since the nurse lived with the family, she took a stand by "refusing to eat in the kitchen with the household help, separating herself and choosing to eat alone.... Mahoney also indicated on her reference that she would eat in the kitchen *alone*" (Darraj, 2005, p. 56). Her devotion to her patients exemplified the words of Florence Nightingale: "The work that tells is the work of the skillful hand, directed by the cool head, and inspired by the loving heart" (Cook, 1913b, p. 384).

Mahoney had the respect of her peers, but was not honored in her lifetime. In 1936, 10 years after her death, the NACGN established the Mary Eliza Mahoney Award for a person who demonstrated outstanding contributions to equal opportunities for minorities in nursing. After the NACGN merged with the American Nurses Association, this award continued and is given at each ANA biennial convention (Carnegie, 1991). Posthumously, Mary Mahoney has received many awards and honors including induction into the ANA Hall of Fame. However, Mahoney would likely be most pleased with two community honors: renaming of the Area 2 Family Life Center in Roxbury to the Mary Eliza Mahoney Family Life Center and a center in her memory established by the Community Health Project in Oklahoma dedicated to provision of health services in isolated communities (Carnegie, 1991).

When the Chi Eta Phi Sorority and the American Nurses Association restored Mary Mahoney's gravesite on August 15, 1973, a speech by Helen Miller clearly described the importance of Mahoney to the nursing profession: "It is significant then that two national nursing organizations have joined with others who are working toward the long-overdue public recognition of this our First Nurse, to accord her the place in History she so richly deserves" (Darraj, 2005, p. 60).

What a wonderful tribute to a true professional!

Implications for Nurse Leaders Today and in the Future
Excellence in Care Delivery

Nurse leaders have numerous challenges and responsibilities, but Mary Mahoney's life demonstrates the most important aspect of nursing leadership: ensuring quality patient care. It is easy to focus on technology, budgets, and reimbursement issues, but the impact of excellence in basic patient care must not be overlooked. Mary Mahoney received accolades from her patients and was recognized for her care as a private duty nurse (Campbell, 2012). She adhered to the precepts of Florence Nightingale, who said

> the symptoms or the sufferings generally considered to be inevitable and incident to the disease are very often not symptoms of the disease at all, but of something quite different—of the want of fresh air, or of light, or of warmth, or of quiet, or of cleanliness, or of punctuality and

care in the administration of diet, of each or of all of these. And this quite as much in private as in hospital nursing. (Nightingale, 1992, p. 5)

Today, patients receive care in many environments, including hospitals, home health agencies, and clinics, and from both private duty nurses and hospital nurses. The importance of basic nursing care has never been more important and must be a priority. Evidence-based strategies create an environment for this and nurse leaders must play a significant role in achieving this priority (Gelinas, 2015). Collaboration must occur "from the bedside to the boardroom" (Gelinas, 2015, p. 4). Interprofessional collaboration must also include the patient and family for basic care to be effective. Basic care must also include the caregivers to ensure a workplace safety culture for them and their patients. Shared decision-making engages staff nurses to champion issues that will enhance patient care delivery. Better nurse staffing has been shown to reduce lengths of stay and complications. Nurse leaders must formulate a business case for nurse staffing that improves clinical quality and safety for patients. They must also increase nurses' efficiency and effectiveness by using Lean techniques to reduce time wasters that keep nurses from patient care. Staff nurses and nurse leaders must work together to create a work environment that "fosters solid basic patient care" (Gelinas, 2015, p. 5). Mary Mahoney delivered such care to her private patients. We can do no less.

— 4 —

Lillian Wald

Urban Crusader

(March 10, 1867–September 1, 1940)

Lillian's Story

Lillian Wald's life changed when she was 22. She was the third of four children of German Jewish parents and grew up in a happy, indulgent family. She was well educated, but undecided about her future. Romances didn't lead to marriage and she wanted to live life on her own terms. Then, she visited her older sister, Julia, who was ill. Julia needed the services of a trained nurse from Bellevue in her home and Lillian was sent to bring the nurse there. The nurse capably cared for Julia and Wald was impressed with her knowledge and skills. She learned how nurses were trained and the scope of their work. Suddenly, Wald had a purpose in her life: to become a trained nurse (Block, 1969).

She met with Irene Sutliffe, the Director of the New York Hospital Training School, and applied for a student position there. Since the course was only open to women 25 and older, Wald took a chance and wrote Julia's birth date on the application (Williams, 1948). Sutliffe was impressed by the new applicant's enthusiasm, but somewhat concerned about her ability to channel her sympathy for the patients into positive actions. In August 1889, Wald began the 18-month training course. Two days later, she heard a man in a locked room yelling that he was hungry. She unlocked the door and took food from the diet kitchen to him. When he had been fed, Wald went to Sutliffe's office to complain about a patient being starved in the hospital. Sutliffe gently explained that the man was recovering from delirium tremens and was offered food earlier that he refused. No one was starving the patient, but the food Wald took was meant for patients on special diets and she shouldn't have taken it without permission. Wald was mortified by her error, but Sutliffe ended the discussion by saying "just the same, I'm glad you fed the old drunk" (Block, 1969, p. 23). Lillian Wald had learned a valuable lesson about channeling her compassion into effective action that she used throughout her nursing career.

Patients loved Lillian Wald and she did everything she could to meet their needs. Her personal growth was evident, but she remained reluctant to enter the operating room. Sutliffe resolved this concern by telling Wald that one of her patients was apprehensive about surgery and needed her support in the OR. Of course, Wald went with the patient. Once there, she was able to assist the surgeon and her fear disappeared (Block, 1969).

After graduation in March 1891, Wald spent a year as a nurse at the New York Juvenile Asylum for children from the ages of 7–14. The experience showed her a system that needed reform and she was frustrated in her efforts to help the children there. She made a difference with a few individuals, but realized that multiple rules and regulations limited her opportunity to support the children (Williams, 1948).

Wald decided at the end of that year to enroll in the Women's Medical College of the New York Infirmary. Although she enjoyed some of the classes, she still wasn't satisfied. She needed to determine her place in the world and studying medicine didn't excite her. Then, she was asked to teach a nursing class in a Jewish Sabbath School on Henry Street. Wald was naïve about the slums and tenements there, but spent a few weeks showing mothers how to make beds and prepare nourishing food. Then, the course of her career and her life changed: A little girl ran into the class and asked for help for her sick mother. Wald accompanied her to a crowded, dirty room where a woman lay bleeding after childbirth. She cared for the mother, cleaned her and the room, and never returned to medical school. At 25, Lillian Wald found her calling in that squalid setting (Williams, 1948; Block, 1965).

Lillian knew these people needed help and set about providing it. She decided that she needed to take nursing service into these homes and to live among the people of the Lower East Side to identify with them socially and establish trust. She began by talking with the philanthropist, Mrs. Solomon (Betty) Loeb, who financed the Henry Street class, and convinced her and her son-in-law, Jacob Schiff, to finance the project. They agreed to contribute $60 per month for Wald and her friend and fellow nurse, Mary Brewster, to live in the neighborhood and supported the venture with funds for medicines, supplies, medical fees, and food for the sick (Williams, 1948).

Wald and Brewster spent a few months in the College Settlement, an organization of women who lived in the neighborhood and stressed self-help through education. This group helped the two nurses acclimate to their new surroundings. Soon it was time to find their own place. They located an apartment on the fifth floor of 27 Jefferson Street that was unique for the area: It had a bathroom! They kept it neat and orderly with a vase of flowers on the table. They also made friends with the janitress and her son, who moved with them two years later to Henry Street (Block, 1969).

The Lower East Side included impoverished immigrants from Ireland, Germany, and Italy, and Jews from Eastern Europe. Housing was poor with high rents. Jobs were difficult to find, and paid meager wages. Many immigrants didn't speak or understand English and the people were afraid of hospitals and visiting nurses, who were ineffective and only interested in converting them. These nurses were viewed as hospital spies (Block, 1969).

Wald and Brewster began their work by establishing relationships with their new neighbors. Both followed the precepts of Florence Nightingale in focusing on cleanliness when providing care (Cook, 1913a, 1913b). They went from apartment to apartment and talked about cleanliness while they bathed and treated children, educated mothers, and enlisted the assistance of all tenants to clean rooms and halls. They also held the janitors responsible for the condition of their buildings. Wald met with the President of the Board of Health and obtained official approval for their work. Each wore a badge that read "Visiting Nurse. Under the Auspices of the Board of Health" (Block, 1969, p. 47). Soon, they were accepted and people came to Jefferson Street all day and into the night seeking help (Block, 1969).

Wald focused on advocating for individuals and improving their health and life. She was now a force in the community and began the first public health nursing service. Although Wald didn't realize it, she was following the advice of Nightingale, who in 1886 wrote that nurses who cared for the sick poor must be "health missionaries" and live within "reach of their work" (Cook, 1913b, p. 253). After their daily duties, she and Brewster were up late writing reports of sickness and unsanitary conditions. They ran interference for sick residents who were cheated out of the little money they had by unscrupulous doctors who then refused treatment. Luckily, other doctors worked with them and accepted their help (Block, 1969).

In 1893, the original project had outgrown the Jefferson Street address. Mary Brewster was ailing and retired and Lillian Wald moved to 265 Henry Street, where a number of nurses and volunteers joined her during the next forty years. Henry Street had trees and a yard where neighborhood children could play and Wald and her team created the first public playground, which she called "the Bunker Hill of playgrounds" (Block, 1969, p. 68). She discovered that numerous children worked in sweatshops, factories, and did piece work at home to help support their families, often when ill with communicable diseases. They had no opportunity for school or play. Wald set out to remedy this by finding volunteers to take children on Sundays to Central or Riverside Park. She kept records of children excluded from school for medical reasons and recommended school nurses to the Board of Health. At first, this idea was too radical, but in 1902, an epidemic of trachoma (infectious eye disease) occurred in the schools and community. Wald put her staff of trained nurses in schools to treat children so they could stay in school. The experiment worked and she challenged the Board of Health to hire school nurses and pay them from public funds. The first school nurse was hired that year and public school nurses spread across the country. Wald also shared an idea with Elizabeth Farrell, a teacher at a nearby school, to develop special education classes without grades for children with physical or mental disabilities. Today, these classes are available throughout the country (Block, 1969).

Wald also provided rooms at the Henry Street Settlement for children to study that were lighted and quiet. Volunteers acted as coaches, books were donated, and time was set aside for small children to learn how to use a library. By 1898, 11 workers lived at Henry Street, accompanied by numerous volunteers, and Lillian Wald was called the Head Worker, a title she would have until her retirement. Breakfast and supper were times for robust discussion and included visitors of all types. Wald used these opportunities to lobby for child labor changes and reform with philanthropists and legislators (Block, 1969).

Wald remembered her own exposure to culture as a child and wanted others to have the same opportunities. She joined the Social Reform Club, which included influential people in education, politics, and literature. While continuing her daily caseload, Wald now was a visible member of commissions to reform the tenements, factories, and support development of a children's bureau by the federal government. This goal was finally realized in 1912. She became knowledgeable about trade unions and participated in founding the National Women's Trade Union, but Wald didn't consider herself a member of any political group. Her focus was on individuals and supporting them to a healthier and better life (Block, 1969).

Wald's life was the Settlement and her neighbors. Even when she traveled around the world in 1910 to look at healthcare issues in other countries, her heart was still in New York's Lower East Side. She also was a proponent for postgraduate courses in public health nursing at Columbia University's Teachers College. While she worked on multiple issues, Wald trusted her colleagues at Henry Street to perform capably with complete independence. There was mutual respect, affection, and communication between everyone there and the team treasured Wald's notes congratulating them for a job well done, called the "L. D. W. degree" (Block, 1969, p. 113).

Henry Street continued to expand, offering social clubs for all age groups, discussion groups, English classes, plays, and music classes with an emphasis on improving their neighbors' lives as well as their health. Lillian Wald's experiment in "district nursing" (Williams, 1948, p. 209) was emulated in settings throughout the world. She insisted that her life had been one of total involvement and fun while dealing with serious issues. Happiness radiated from Wald and, when Albert Einstein met her in 1938 two years before her death, his parting words were "I want to thank you for your smile" (Block, 1946, p. 172). It was an apt tribute for a nursing crusader who truly changed the world.

Implications for Nurse Leaders Today and in the Future
Living Cultural Diversity

Lillian Wald's approach to diversity was unique—learn about a needy, immigrant population by living in their midst, sharing their problems, and preparing them for a better life (Williams, 1948). Today's nurse leaders realize the importance of diversity and know that race and ethnic background influence health outcomes (Wesley, 2015). Many healthcare facilities hire diversity specialists and plan celebrations around holidays specific to local cultures. That's a start, but doesn't go far enough. Nurse leaders must educate themselves and other health team members about the health practices of the populations—racial, ethnic, religious, sexual, and cultural—in their service areas (Wesley, 2015). They can promote ongoing discussion with members of these communities and ensure advocacy for these practices in the healthcare environment. They also can learn from Lillian Wald, who carefully selected the members of Henry Street based on their ability to relate to their neighbors along with their skills. She trusted their caring as well as their competence (Block, 1969). Today's nurse leaders must hire based on competence, but with a focus on enabling these employees to develop "personal and organizational diversity leadership skills" (Wesley, 2015, p. 52). It is imperative that nurse leaders seek diversity in hiring to reflect population demographics. They must also enhance their own knowledge of diversity by subscribing to the National Center for Healthcare Leadership's core leadership competencies: "identify and manage the impact of formative life experiences; expand one's worldview that embraces key diversity dimensions; accept and manage one's own implicit biases; self-monitor and adjust one's communication style; and utilize cognitive reframing to change one's behavior" (Wesley, 2015, p. 52). Lillian Wald practiced each of these behaviors. Today's nurse leaders can do no less.

Leveraging Managed Care

Today's nurse leaders live in a managed care world, but many don't realize that managed care is not a 20th-century norm that has extended into the 21st century. Lillian Wald was one of the first to leverage managed care to benefit her neighbors and clients. When she saw that poor immigrants were paying insurance premiums they couldn't afford for health care, Wald made an appointment in 1909 with the medical director of Metropolitan Life Insurance Company to propose that the company provide free nursing services for working class customers. The idea was a novel one at the time, but she convinced him that sending nurses promptly where needed would result in fewer claims and better health for their clients. Initially Met Life employed Henry Street nurses to care for their policyholders on the Lower East Side. The reduction in sickness and mortality was phenomenal. After that, Met Life set up its own visiting nurse service department and extended this approach to nearly all policyholders in the United States and Canada. Their nursing department provided clients with booklets on health and hygiene and provided health education to millions of people (Block, 1969). The idea of nursing care bought and paid for through insurance spread to encompass today's managed care because of Lillian Wald's idea to benefit both her neighbors and Metropolitan Life.

Today, nurse leaders must also leverage managed care to benefit their patients and their organizations. They need to promote wellness, not just treat illness. Many hospitalized patients have Medicare as their primary insurance provider and the Hospital Readmission Reduction Program of the Affordable Care Act financially penalizes hospitals for preventable readmissions within 30 days of discharge (Nelson & Rosenthal, 2015). Nurse leaders play an important role in preventing these readmissions by increasing their staff members' collaboration with nurse case managers. As Lillian Wald's Henry Street nurses promoted health for Met Life policyholders, today's nurse case managers promote health and reduce preventable readmissions starting when the patient arrives on the unit. Nurse leaders must ensure that clinical staff members support the case manager's role in

> *appropriately determining the patient's readiness for discharge; compiling a comprehensive and accurate discharge summary; helping to determine an appropriate post-discharge care setting; coordinating care with multiple settings and providers; involving the patient and family caregivers in the plan of care; and conducting post-discharge follow-up phone calls. (Nelson & Rosenthal, 2015, p. 18)*

Lillian Wald's radical idea has become an everyday occurrence and nurse leaders must continue to leverage managed care to benefit their patients and their organizations now and in the future.

— 5 —

Mary Adelaide Nutting
Nurse Scholar
(November 1, 1858–October 3, 1948)

Adelaide's Story

Mary Adelaide Nutting was the eldest daughter in a large Canadian family of limited means. Adelaide took advantage of the education opportunities available to her to study French, music, literature, piano, and art design. When her mother became ill, she realized how unprepared she was to deal with illness and death: "I am convinced, I must learn how to take care of my family" (Marshall, 1972, p. 28).

Nutting read about Florence Nightingale and wrote a paper on her for a class. She sent for a copy of Nightingale's *Notes on Nursing*. Nutting learned that there were hospitals in the United States using Nightingale's training methods and that she could receive lodging and a small wage while studying and working at a training school for nurses. Since this would solve her financial problems, she decided to apply at one of these schools (Marshall, 1972).

Nutting first applied to Bellevue in New York City. Then, she read an article about a new hospital and training school at Johns Hopkins in Baltimore. This facility was more modern and progressive than other hospitals and there were three Canadians on staff there, including Isabel Hampton, the principal of the Training School for Nurses. Nutting was 31 and healthy when she entered Hopkins and that was an advantage for the long hours probationers devoted to work, study, and classes. On her first day, she was assigned to Ward H, women's gynecology, and told to observe that day and do as she was told. After that, she was to do everything without being asked. There were few textbooks and no library. She and her classmates were expected to buy or borrow *Gray's Anatomy* and Martin's *Human Body*. Some head nurses also owned a copy of Clara Weeks's *Textbook of Nursing*, the first nursing textbook (Marshall, 1972).

Nutting entered a world of obedience to authority and took notes on physicians' lectures. Students' notebooks were graded on neatness, accuracy, and completeness. She notes that "lecture books became the bane of our existence. We came home too fatigued to write and fill in the gaps" (Marshall, 1972, p. 40). Her first month's pay of $8 bought a copy of the *Textbook of Nursing* to prepare her for written, oral, and practical exams.

Her first attempt at writing was when the *Trained Nurse and Hospital Review* offered prizes for stories about typhoid fever cases and their treatment in November 1890. Nutting's essay won $10 and she was published in March 1891. She graduated that year and, after four months of private duty, returned to Hopkins as a head nurse. The following year, she served as acting superintendent during the superintendent's vacation and became assistant superintendent in 1893. She enjoyed that role because it offered her the opportunity to teach (Marshall, 1972).

In July 1894, Isabel Hampton married and the Board designated Nutting as acting superintendent, but offered her $300 less per year than her predecessor. She refused to accept the position, but offered to stay on until someone was found. Her work was excellent and in September, she officially became Superintendent of Nurses and Principal of the Training School at Hopkins at the same salary as Hampton. The Board agreed to give her a leave to tour hospitals in the United States and Great Britain as part of a committee to investigate a three-year program and eight-hour plan for students. On her return from Glasgow and London, Nutting focused on establishing a three-year nursing course with only one class admitted annually. She also focused on establishing an eight-hour day for students and using the third year for education about administration. In her words, "less work, more education is needed" (Marshall, 1972, p. 72).

Nutting did research and statistical analysis to determine the effect of reduction of work hours for students and presented her results in her first national address at the 3rd Annual Meeting of the American Society of Superintendents. This speech established her as a potential leader within nursing and resulted in her appointment as president for 1897. This position enabled her to advocate for fewer and better training schools for nurses. She continued to fulfill her role at Hopkins, focusing on a new curriculum, discipline, and maintaining standards (Marshall, 1972).

Nutting became well known for her outstanding committee work and careful data-driven studies about nursing education. She and Isabel Hampton Robb developed a postgraduate course for nurse administrators at Teachers College of Columbia University in 1899. This course, called Hospital Economics, would change nursing education dramatically and set the direction for the rest of Adelaide Nutting's professional career. She began teaching classes in the Hospital Economics course in the early 1900s and ensured that it remained an advanced education program. Her motivation was a college of nursing and, with the support of the superintendents, the Carnegie Foundation was asked to finance the Teachers College graduate nursing program (Marshall, 1972).

Adelaide Nutting and other nurse leaders also saw the need for a nursing journal and the *American Journal of Nursing* was born in 1900. In 1904, she expressed her thoughts about nursing education succinctly in the October 1904 edition: "Nursing is one of the few branches of education where more emphasis is placed on age, height, weight, and freedom from family ties and less exacting about educational qualifications" (Marshall, 1972, p. 121). She would become a prolific writer of papers, editorials, and books for the rest of her life.

After 11 years at Johns Hopkins, Nutting decided to focus her future on collegiate nursing education as Chair of Hospital Administration at Teachers College. Her numerous accomplishments at Hopkins included lowering the admission age to 21, a preparatory course, non-pay for students and student scholarships, eight-hour days for students, and a three-year nursing course that included public health services. Her commencement day address in 1906 reflected her future goals:

> *We are in urgent need of nursing schools founded on a separate and independent basis in which the course of study and training will be*

complete, each hospital contributing what it fairly can as a field for teaching and receiving of the student, what she must necessarily give in obtaining her practical training and experience. The formation of such a school is the next step forward. (Marshall, 1972, p. 138)

A year later, Nutting spent time in England that included a half hour with Florence Nightingale in her home. Nightingale was interested in American nursing and seemed "wonderfully sympathetic as if an unquenchable spirit still shone in her eyes and filled her voice" (Marshall, 1972, p. 150). When Nutting rose to leave, Nightingale said, "No, tell me more" (Marshall, 1972, p. 150). Nightingale asked her to come again and Nutting treasured that experience the rest of her life.

In September 1907, Adelaide Nutting began her work at Teachers College and enhanced her own knowledge by studying teaching methods and techniques, psychology and social sciences, and self-disciplined reading to keep up with advances in medicine and nursing. She collaborated with Lillian Wald to provide instruction on public health and concentrated on developing a variety of courses to complement Hospital Economics. An endowment enabled the creation of a separate Department of Nursing and Health to offer classes in administration, nursing education, and public health. Adelaide Nutting became the first nurse to attain professional rank in any university (Marshall, 1972).

Nutting's reputation as a nurse educator and administrator resulted in a request by the U.S. Office of Education for a report on the status of training schools for nurses. She completed the first comprehensive study of nursing education in the United States—and perhaps in the world—in 1911, a work that was widely cited (Marshall, 1972).

During her tenure, Teachers College became a graduate school that awarded bachelor's and master's degrees to students from all over the world, with a faculty actively engaged in research activities. In an editorial for the Johns Hopkins *Alumnae Magazine*, Nutting wrote:

The education of nurses passes over into a new era. It is because for the first time in history the education of nurses is accorded the status and powers which are recognized in the conduct and development of other forms of professional education. (Marshall, 1972, p. 287)

Her numerous papers and presentations enabled her to promote endowments for nursing education and she received numerous honors and awards during her lifetime, including an honorary Master of Arts degree from Yale and her portrait in gown and hood hung on the walls of Teachers College—the first woman to receive this accolade.

Mary Adelaide Nutting never amassed wealth, but was respected and loved by her peers, students, and colleagues in all disciplines. In 1944, the National League for Nursing Education (forerunner of the National League for Nursing) created the Mary Adelaide Nutting Award for outstanding contributions to nursing. This award recognized and encouraged leadership in nursing education and research. The first recipient was Mary Adelaide Nutting at a ceremony in her New York apartment (Marshall, 1972).

The most fitting tribute to Mary Adelaide Nutting came from the President of the National League for Nursing Education: "You have been the torch which has shown the way and we are eager to follow on" (Marshall, 1972, p. 351).

Implications for Nurse Leaders Today and in the Future
Promoting Collegiate Education

Mary Adelaide Nutting moved nursing education from servitude to the hospital to a respected school in a university setting (Marshall, 1972). An IOM report states: "Nurses should achieve higher levels of education and training through an improved education system that promotes seamless academic progression" (IOM, 2011, p. 163). Nurse leaders play a pivotal role in promoting collegiate education for themselves and their staff nurses. A goal of increasing the percentage of BSN-prepared nurses to 80% by 2020 has been adopted by numerous healthcare organizations (IOM, 2011, p. 173). The need for APRNs, nurse faculty members, and nurse researchers continues to grow and these are also identified as critical education needs (IOM, 2011).

Nurse leaders must promote revenue sources for both undergraduate and graduate education. They must be knowledgeable about tuition assistance, loan repayment programs, available grants, and community resources, such as scholarships. Representatives of local and regional nursing programs can be scheduled for career fairs so current staff members can discuss admission requirements, course requirements, time commitments, and program costs with them. Employees may also explore accredited online programs with encouragement from their nurse leaders. Conversations about work assignments and flexible scheduling must occur prior to starting the course (Sherrod, 2015).

Nurse leaders must consider their own educational needs and use the same "planning, negotiating, scheduling, prioritizing, organizing, and triaging skills" (Sherrod, 2015, p. 14) they encourage their staff members to use in establishing a sound personal education pathway. This approach is an opportunity to achieve higher levels of nursing education and prepare nurses to function collaboratively in a complex healthcare environment (IOM, 2011). Adelaide Nutting would encourage today's nurses to continue their academic progression as she did college graduates completing nurses training in 1918:

> About thirty distinct branches of nursing, many of them in the big new field of public health nursing, are calling them. College women are wanted because their previous education facilitates intensive training and more rapid advancement to posts of urgent need. (Marshall, 1972, p. 236)

Those words were true then and remain so today and in the future.

~ 6 ~

Lavinia Lloyd Dock

Activist and Historian

(February 26, 1858–April 17, 1956)

Lavinia's Story

Lavinia Dock was a force to be reckoned with, both in nursing and in life. She was one of six children in a prosperous Pennsylvania family and was well educated for her era. She enjoyed reading and music, especially the piano. Reading a magazine article inspired her to consider a nursing career (American Association for the History of Nursing [AAHN], 2007b). She entered the Training School for Nurses at Bellevue Hospital in 1884 and graduated as a nurse in 1886. Her first nursing position was as night superintendent at Bellevue and her experiences included disaster relief during a yellow fever epidemic in Jacksonville, Florida (1888), and at the Johnstown Flood of 1889 (AAHN, 2007b).

In November 1890, Dock became an assistant to Isabel Hampton, the principal of the Training School for Nurses at Johns Hopkins Hospital in Baltimore (Marshall, 1972). In this role, she conducted classes for the middle class and junior class of students. Lavinia Dock began a journey at Hopkins that would change American nursing.

Textbooks were limited. Many physicians were ignorant about the drugs they prescribed and nurses often found discrepancies in dosages for administration. Dock decided to remedy this situation and wrote a textbook for nurses called *Materia Medica* that described different drugs, their dosages, and indications/contraindications. The textbook was so complete that many readers were physicians seeking to enrich their knowledge of medications (Marshall, 1972).

This textbook would be the first of many books written by Lavinia Dock in her career. She became superintendent of the Illinois Training School in Chicago in 1893 and her involvement in professional nursing organizations began that year. Her involvement in the founding of the Society of Superintendents of Training Schools resulted in her selection as secretary. She was a founder of the Nurses' Associated Alumnae (forerunner of ANA) and the International Council of Nurses, where she served as secretary for 22 years (AAHN, 2007b).

Dock joined Lillian Wald's Henry Street Settlement in 1896 and spent the next 16 years there. She had a gift for languages and learned enough of the immigrants' languages on the Lower East Side to communicate successfully. Her sensitivity, nursing skills, and empathy endeared her to neighborhood residents. She also continued to lecture at the Teachers College of Columbia University's graduate nursing program on the "History of Nursing and Hospitals" (Marshall, 1972, p. 153).

Dock's interests included social activism, writing, and self-regulation of the nursing profession. The early 20th century was a time of the birth of unions and the suffrage movement for women's rights. Lavinia Dock was active in both movements. She walked picket lines and asked the 1913 ANA Convention to support the union movement. Dock helped found a local chapter of the United Garment Workers of America and encouraged workers to join trade unions. She picketed numerous times for women's suffrage and was jailed three times in 1917 for participating in confrontational demonstrations. She also was a crusader against venereal disease and her book, *Hygiene & Morality*, was published in 1910 and demanded elimination of the double standard of morality for men and women. This book also promoted the elimination of prostitution, self-control for men, and the right to vote for women (AAHN, 2007b).

Lavinia Dock was fascinated by the history of nursing and, except for Nightingale's writings to her nurses at the Nightingale School, there was little information available about nursing history (Nightingale, 2012). Dock set out to remedy this deficiency. In 1907, she collaborated with Adelaide Nutting on the first two volumes of the *History of Nursing*, a comprehensive review of nursing throughout the centuries. Then, she traveled in Europe to secure more source materials for the third volume and completed the third and fourth volumes herself in 1912. Dock collaborated with Isabel Stewart on *A Short History of Nursing* and with Sarah E. Pickett on the *History of American Red Cross Nursing*. These works established Lavinia Dock as the foremost nursing historian (Lavinia Dock Collection, n.d.). The American Association for the History of Nursing has recognized her with the Lavinia L. Dock Award for Exemplary Historical Research and Writing (AAHN, 2007a).

Dock's interest in nursing history and its value for the nursing profession was aptly expressed in the fourth edition of *A Short History of Nursing*:

> *The nurse or teacher who knows only her own time and surroundings is not only deprived of an unfailing source of interest; she may also be unable to estimate and judge correctly the current events whose tendency is likely to affect her own career. We must know how our work of nursing arose; what lines it has followed and under what direction it has developed best. Possessing this knowledge each one may help to guide and influence its future in harmony with its historical mission. (Dock & Stewart, 1938, pp. 3–4)*

In addition to social activism and writing, Dock's greatest contribution to nursing was in her desire to "establish a recognized standard of professional education" (Dock, 1900, p. 9) and secure laws to ensure nursing control of the profession. This was vital to resolve the exploitation of students, long hours, lack of uniformity in training standards, and elimination of six-week and correspondence schools of nursing. She advocated state organizations for nurses, salaried positions for graduate nurses in hospitals, postgraduate work in specialty hospitals, and availability of specialized training for students (Marshall, 9172; Dock, 1900).

Her concern for "having no recognized standard of work or requirements" (Marshall, 1972, p. 79) was met and Lavinia Dock's work is reflected in today's nurse practice acts and licensing examinations. She truly was a force to be reckoned with in nursing and in life.

Implications for Nurse Leaders Today and in the Future
Legislative Advocacy

Lavinia Dock believed in causes and the legislative process. Her support for the Nineteenth Amendment and state organization and registration for nurses demonstrated the success of legislation (Marshall, 1972). However, she also knew that laws must be enforced and revised as practice changes occur (Dock, 1900). Although Florence Nightingale would not have agreed with Dock about the importance of registration for nurses (Cook, 1913b), both would have supported the idea "that nursing was an art, and must be raised to the status of a trained profession" (Cook, 1913a, p. 445). In the United States, laws safeguarded the progression of that profession.

Today's nurse leaders must ensure that laws regulating nursing practice meet current and future standards for the profession. They must be knowledgeable about their state's nurse practice act and alert to proposed changes, particularly the role of the state boards of nursing in interpreting and enforcing the act (ANA, 2012). These acts are readily available online and define nurses' responsibilities, qualifications for practice, and the activities and services performed by nurses (ANA, 2012).

According to the Institute of Medicine, "emphasis is placed on advanced practice registered nurses (APRNs), including their roles in chronic disease management and increased access to primary care, and the regulatory barriers preventing them from taking on these roles" (2011, p. 86). Moving in this direction will require changes in nurse practice acts to reflect these changes in their scope of practice (ANA, 2012).

Nurse leaders also have responsibility to ensure their staff nurses practice to the extent of their skills and knowledge and this requires them to understand their state's nurse practice act. They should be able to access the act easily and receive education about proposed changes and their ability to provide input to the state board of nursing about nursing practice standards (ANA, 2012). Leaders can use a variety of approaches to provide this information: unit meetings, written communication, education activities, group discussion, and electronic messaging. Nurses need to remember that legislation regulating the nursing profession is not "just one effort, but continuous efforts for the rest of time" (Dock, 1900).

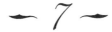

Annie Warburton Goodrich
Pacifist and Patriot

(February 6, 1866–December 31, 1954)

Annie's Story

Annie Goodrich came from a distinguished family. Her ancestor was the second president of Harvard and her grandfather, Dr. John S. Butler, was a pioneer in psychiatry in New England (Koch, 1951; Yost, 1955). In 1880, Goodrich's father transferred to London to supervise development of the Equitable Life Assurance company in Europe. she attended school in London and Paris, where she developed a fondness for French cuisine and a fluent command of the French language. She also became interested in different types of people and acquired a broad educational foundation.

When Goodrich was 17, the family returned to Hartford, Connecticut, and took her grandparents into their home during their last illnesses. She was close to her grandfather and shared in his care prior to his death (Yost, 1955). Her mother hired a graduate nurse who was uninformed about nursing techniques and unable to provide good nursing care. Goodrich thought how much more effective the nurse could be if she had the general education of a refined person to gain the patient's confidence and trust with understanding and empathy. She understood that devotion and a desire to help the sick were not enough for a nurse to care for patients.

Goodrich realized that nurses required technical competence, knowledge about the reasons for their activities, and the social experience to adapt to any situation for the patient's benefit (Koch, 1951).

Nursing interested Goodrich as an opportunity to be self-supporting and independent although she did not see nursing as a calling. In 1891, she was accepted at the New York Hospital's nurse training school and demonstrated the ability to become a skilled nurse. She was gentle and reassuring to patients and accepted responsibility for their care. Goodrich also showed her ability to deal with emergencies when she was a student head nurse in a men's ward during a smallpox outbreak. She and two assistants were isolated with their patients and one of the assistants developed the disease. Goodrich and her remaining assistant handled the epidemic so well that the hospital Board gave each of them a commendation and $50 (Yost, 1955).

Goodrich's straightforward approach to problems and use of evidence would endure throughout her career and showed when she was in a three-month rotation at the Sloane Maternity Hospital. When the medical superintendent complained because nursing students didn't complete their assignments in a timely fashion, she did a time study that revealed that the expectations for 11 hours of care really took 17 hours! Although no change occurred, Goodrich always approached problems clearly and with proof (Koch, 1951).

After graduation, Goodrich was offered graduate head nurse positions and accepted one in the men's surgical ward until May 1893. Then, she accepted the position of superintendent of nurses at the New York Postgraduate Hospital and began her administrative responsibilities. This hospital had an independent nurse training school and Goodrich, who was responsible for hospital nurses and patient care, had no official role in students' education. That didn't stop her from holding weekly "class nights" (Koch, 1951, p. 27) at the nurses' residence. One of the students described her thusly:

> She was a born teacher and taught her pupils not from classroom and lecture only, but by personal demonstration on the wards. She imbued her pupils with her own passionate interest in the intelligent and tender care of the sick and a never-failing devotion to the medical profession and the hospital. (Koch, 1951, p. 27)

By 1895, the cost of a separate training school caused the Board to take control of the school as part of the facility. Goodrich became superintendent of both nursing and the training school. She reorganized the curriculum and fostered a progressive education program. Textbooks materialized and she campaigned for better-qualified students. Goodrich's insistence that only students with high school diplomas be admitted achieved this result during the seven years she was there (Koch, 1951).

Annie Goodrich became a dynamic administrator who collaborated with the Board to create a school with high standards and established sound relationships with physicians. She saw medicine and nursing as separate professions that depended on each other and were equal in status. In more than 50 years as a nurse executive, Annie Goodrich demonstrated her belief in the dignity and worth of the nursing profession without offending other disciplines (Yost, 1955).

Between 1900 and 1910, Goodrich served as director and superintendent of training schools for St. Luke's Hospital, the New York Hospital, and Bellevue Hospital. During these years, she created a sense of freedom where authority was respected, not feared. Discipline was fair and students were expected to think for themselves. She was approachable, a good listener, and never appeared rushed when students sought her out. Since she had capably dealt with housekeeping issues on wards during her tenure in these facilities, Goodrich became interested in hospital design. Following the example of Florence Nightingale, she advocated window placement for patients, hospital planning for expansion, availability of elevators or dumb-waiters for linen and dietary departments, inclusion of clothing closets for patients, and arrangements for heating and disinfection (Cook, 1913a; Yost, 1955).

At Bellevue (the first Nightingale training school in the United States), Annie Goodrich created affiliations with other facilities for student training. Such affiliations later became accepted avenues to provide well-rounded education for student nurses in small or specialized schools. She also recognized the need for postgraduate courses for nurses and arranged a nine-month general course and a three-month certificate course in 1908. In 1909, 100 nurses enrolled in these courses and 60 certificates were awarded. Participants enrolled in either preparation for executive positions or in preparation for general nursing. Goodrich remained active in professional nursing organizations and served as chair of the Committee on Hospital Economics for the Superintendents' Society. In this role, she was involved in planning the Hospital Economics Course for postgraduate study at Columbia University (Yost, 1955).

She arranged for probationers to be admitted at specific times of the year with a three-month probationary period that was completed by practical and written exams.

In 1910, the position of Inspector of Nurses' Training Schools in New York State was open. There was pressure to make this civil service position a political appointment for a non-nurse. Many schools were exploiting students and others were poorly run and provided inferior education. These schools were suspicious of any inspection and only a skilled, proficient nurse would raise the standards of nursing education to a professional level. Only one nurse had the qualifications, experience, and vision to win cooperation of training school superintendents in this complex role—Annie Warburton Goodrich. She succeeded beyond anyone's expectations. Her inclusive approach and emphasis on higher standards resulted in visionary and workable recommendations and her accurate, honest reports of training school conditions provided the impetus for change in nurses' training. In 1912, 90% of women calling themselves nurses had no education or had attended correspondence schools (Koch, 1951). In 1913, Goodrich asked the Superintendents' Society to promote legal requirements that would establish standards for nurses' training. These requirements included requiring four years of high school for admission, minimum standards of professional education, three-year course length, inspections of schools, and mandatory state registration of nurses. She made her point by saying "We are knocking at the doors of the college.... We will never render our full service to the community until our place is found in the university" (Yost, 1955, p. 67).

Goodrich found her place at the university level in 1914 when she was appointed Assistant Professor of Nursing Education at Teachers College, a position she would hold for four years. She was elected the president of ANA in 1916 and Lillian Wald asked her at the end of that year to become the general director of the Henry Street Settlement. For 1917, Goodrich held both these full-time positions capably, succeeding in improving hours and salaries for the Settlement's nurses and planning a program for student nurses to affiliate at Henry Street for public health nursing. She wanted to prepare all nurses for preventative health as well as promoting public health nursing (Yost, 1955).

During her years at Bellevue, Goodrich became a dedicated pacifist and suffragist. In 1918, this committed pacifist was asked to be Chief Inspecting Nurse of Army Hospitals and join the Surgeon General's Office. The problem she faced was how to train enough nurses to meet all emergencies. She organized her staff for inspections and reports and convinced the secretary of war to approve her plan for a school of nursing to meet Army needs. In May, she was appointed Dean of the Army School of Nursing. In five months, 1,600 student nurses were sent to hospitals at 31 training camps with a director and staff of supervisors and teachers at each camp. Every student had completed four years of high school and many had attended college. Her Army School of Nursing continued after the war until financial problems eliminated it in 1931 (Koch, 1951).

In 1919, she returned to civilian life and resumed her two full-time jobs, while participating in state, national, and international nursing organizations. In recognition of her service, Annie Goodwich was awarded the Distinguished Service Medal 4 years later. In 1923, Goodrich served on a small committee to create plans for a school of nursing at Yale University. This school was equal with the schools of other professions at Yale and Annie Warburton Goodrich was appointed the first Dean and Professor of Nursing Education, a post she held for 11 years. During that time, she developed the school into the Yale Graduate School of Nursing, demanding 4 years of college for admission, and granting MSN degrees. Her expertise and dedication ensured that nursing found its place in the university setting.

Goodrich's finest tribute may be in the following statement by Edna Yost in 1955:

> *Here then, is the story of a nurse who believes that the public has the right to expect professional nursing care whenever and wherever this is needed. It is the story of an educator who believes that 'knowledge is more than power; it is a definite responsibility.' It is the story of a pioneer who blazed new trails that others might follow without fear. It is the story of a citizen who, although a devout pacifist, put on her country's uniform to assist with the war effort. It is the story of the nursing profession—how it has fought, and finally won, its battle for equal standing with other professions. (Yost, 1955, pp. 148–149)*

Annie Goodrich would certainly approve this sentiment.

Implications for Nurse Leaders Today and in the Future
Health Promotion

Annie Goodrich believed in the preparation of all nurses in the field of preventive medicine. In her words, "our goal is the healthy individual. Our goal means a better world" (Yost, 1955, p. 76). This goal reflects Florence Nightingale's doctrine that "nursing the well" (Cook, 1913a, p. 452) is even more important than caring for the sick. Today's nurse leaders in acute care must focus beyond the walls of the facility when coordinating patient care. Promoting health across the continuum is a goal in today's complex healthcare system. Nurses are essential to reducing "lengths of stay, cost per case, adverse events" (Fitzpatrick, 2015, p. 3) as well as "preventing readmissions and ensuring that patients successfully navigate the many hand-offs that occur during their stay" (Fitzpatrick, 2015, p. 3).

For nurses to meet these expectations, their leaders must ensure that they are able to spend time with patients and families, helping them achieve goals for wellness and encouraging their participation in care. The nurse's presence is integral to the patient's progress and ability to function outside the hospital setting. Nurse leaders must also be knowledgeable about the community resources available for patients to prevent readmissions and ensure their safety. Nurse leaders must share this knowledge with their nurses "as they manage and coordinate the patient's care to ensure safe passage through the care-delivery system" (Fitzpatrick, 2015, p. 3).

Involvement in community health and wellness initiatives is also important for both nurses and nurse leaders. *Nursing: Scope and Standards of Practice* has a standard on health teaching and health promotion. To meet this standard, nurse leaders are obligated to promote education of community members by engaging "consumer alliance and advocacy groups in health teaching and health promotion activities for healthcare consumers" (ANA, 2015b, p. 65). Then Annie Goodrich's goal and Florence Nightingale's doctrine will be realized today and in the future.

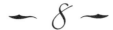

Isabel Hampton Robb

Nursing Visionary

(August 26, 1859–April 15, 1910)

Isabel's Story

Isabel "Addie" Hampton did not plan to be a nurse. One of seven children in a Canadian family, she learned as a child that "duty and work always came before inclination" (Cameron, McIsaac, Dock, Nutting, & Robb, 1910, p. 9). At 17, she went to a nearby town to teach in a public school for $300/year. For the next four years, Hampton stayed with a family in nearby St. Catharine's and had some private lessons in Latin and German. Her teaching certificate covered three years, but the school board contracted her for an additional year. At the end of that time, she was required to take a difficult examination to continue teaching and couldn't pass it. Her choice of a nursing career resulted from a discussion with two of her fellow teachers who sent for a blank application from the Bellevue Training School. They decided to continue teaching for the security it provided, but Hampton filled in the application and mailed it. Later, her friends decided to become nurses and eventually found employment in important nursing positions (Cameron et al., 1910).

Hampton was accepted at Bellevue's Training School. The assistant superintendent recognized the potential of this student who would become "the greatest teacher of nurses in her time" (Cameron et al., 1910, p. 11). Her classmates were not as fond of Hampton. She wanted to learn all she could and followed up on topics by questioning doctors and reading every book she could find. Her thirst for education meant that she wasn't as rapid as her classmates in performing activities of daily living for patients. Other students were faster, but none was more thorough. Hampton enjoyed her training experiences and always fulfilled her duties at her own pace (Cameron et al., 1910).

After graduation, Hampton worked for a short time in the Woman's Hospital in New York and then spent two years at St. Paul's House in Rome. After her return, she became superintendent of the Illinois Training School for Nurses. This was her first leadership experience and her charm and dignity endeared her to her probationers. Hampton was the first superintendent to establish a grading system to assess students' competency. She also affiliated with Presbyterian Hospital to provide students with the opportunity to care for private patients (Cameron et al., 1910). Today, such affiliations are common, but they were not contemplated in the 1880s.

After three years, the training school was thriving and Hampton was ready for a new challenge. She moved to Baltimore in 1889 and began organizing the Johns Hopkins Training School for Nurses there. The next five years established Isabel Hampton as a force in nursing education (Draper, 1902). Her influence gained respect for her students in the community and she demanded the same respect for her own authority. Hampton focused on establishing uniform standards for nursing education and her visionary leadership created a training school that was a role model for others (Cameron et al., 1910). During this time, she wrote a textbook that became a guidebook for nursing practice: *Nursing: Its Principles and Practices* (Cameron et al., 1910).

Hampton's genius and enthusiasm caused her to envision future nursing growth through development of a national organization that would guide the profession into the future. She saw future graduate nurses prepared for leadership in the standardized Hospital Economics course at Teachers College. Isabel Hampton was a dynamic leader with a natural aptitude for organization. Her energy and joy were evident in her five years at Hopkins (Cameron et al., 1910).

In June 1894, Isabel Hampton did something that was unheard of for nurse leaders of her generation. She resigned her position at Hopkins to accept the proposal of Dr. Hunter Robb, an obstetrician/gynecologist at Hopkins. Her colleagues were shocked and believed she would leave nursing after her marriage. That never happened. Isabel Hampton married Dr. Robb on July 11, 1894, at St. Margaret's Church in Westminster, England. She carried flowers sent to her by Florence Nightingale and accompanied her husband to Cleveland, Ohio, where she would have two sons and continue her work on nursing organization (Draper, 1902; Cameron et al., 1910).

Many of Hampton Robb's greatest professional achievements occurred after her marriage. She was instrumental in founding the first national nursing organization, the Society of Superintendents of Training Schools, and she served as the first president of the Associated Alumnae of the United States. She advocated for lengthening the training courses for nurses from two years to three years, adopting an eight-hour day for students, and eliminating the stipend to students and using that money to obtain equipment and library books for them. These ideas are accepted today, but were radical in Hampton Robb's time. Her foresight would guide the education of nurses in the 20th century and her emphasis on organization and uniform standards enhanced the growth of the nursing profession (Cameron et al., 1910).

Isabel Hampton Robb's commitment to nursing was exemplified in the success of nursing organizations and her practical papers and speeches about nursing education and practice, including the first book on ethics for nurses, *Nursing Ethics* (Draper, 1902). Her contributions to the profession were numerous and ongoing until her untimely death in a streetcar accident in 1910. Her husband shared her unpublished notes after her death and they reveal her love and engagement in nursing:

> *I have always believed that there are few, if any, occupations engaged in by women that will hold the same promise for a full and useful and happy life... as does that of the trained nurse when once nursing has been placed upon the proper footing and its deserts and needs have been met. (Cameron et al., 1910, p. 26)*

Implications for Nurse Leaders Today and in the Future
Ethical Behavior

In the first book on nursing ethics, Isabel Hampton Robb made a statement that is applicable to today's nursing practice:

> *The scientific and educational side is important and should certainly receive its due consideration, but none the less should each nurse see to it that the spirit of love for the work's sake is fostered and developed, in order that we may have a professional code of ethics of an eminently practical and helpful nature. (Robb, 1912, p. 38)*

Throughout *Nursing Ethics*, Hampton Robb delineates the nurse's duty to her patients, her colleagues, physicians, and herself. This mirrors today's *Code of Ethics for Nurses* and Nightingale's *Notes on Nursing* (ANA, 2015a; Nightingale, 1992). What does this mean for today's nurse leaders?

Nurses have become better educated and more technologically proficient since the time of Nightingale and Robb, but one thing has not changed: the requirement for ethical practice. Nurse leaders must ensure that they and their nurse colleagues apply the Provisions of the current *Code of Ethics for Nurses* in their daily performance. For this to occur, they must know the Provisions of the Code and be able to readily access it during their work time. This may mean the nurse leader's advocacy for the Code to be available on the facility intranet for 24/7 viewing by nurses. Discussion about the Code in staff meetings will keep it visible within the organization. Most of all, the nurse leader must demonstrate adherence to the tenets of the Code to role model these behaviors to other nurse colleagues. The following Provisions must be instilled in every nurse's clinical practice:

> "*Provision 1*—The nurse practices with compassion and respect for the inherent dignity, worth, and unique attributes of every person" (ANA, 2015a, p. 1).

> "*Provision 2*—The nurse's primary commitment is to the patient, whether an individual, family, group, community, or population" (ANA, 2015a, p. 5).

> "*Provision 3*—The nurse promotes, advocates for, and protects the rights, health, and safety of patients" (ANA, 2015a, p. 9).

> "*Provision 4*—The nurse has the authority, accountability, and responsibility for nursing practice; makes decisions; and takes

action consistent with the obligation to promote health and to provide optimal care" (ANA, 2015a, p. 15).

"Provision 5—The nurse owes the same duties to self as to others, including the responsibility to promote health and safety, preserve wholeness of character and integrity, maintain competence, and continue personal and professional growth" (ANA, 2015a, p. 19).

"Provision 6—The nurse, through individual and collective effort, establishes, maintains, and improves the ethical environment of the work setting and conditions of employment that are conducive to safe, quality health care" (ANA, 2015a, p. 23).

"Provision 7—The nurse, in all roles and settings, advances the profession through research and scholarly inquiry, professional standards development, and the generation of both nursing and health policy" (ANA, 2015a, p. 27).

"Provision 8—The nurse collaborates with other health professionals and the public to protect human rights, promote health diplomacy, and reduce health disparities" (ANA, 2015a, p. 31).

"Provision 9—The profession of nursing, collectively through its professional organizations, must articulate nursing values, maintain the integrity of the profession, and integrate principles of social justice into nursing and health policy" (ANA, 2015a, p. 35).

When Isabel Hampton Robb started the first professional nursing organizations and wrote the first book on nursing ethics, she established the path that has led to today's ethical nursing practice. It is the accountability and responsibility of today's nurse leaders to advance that practice in the future.

$$\sim 9 \sim$$

Mary Breckinridge

Pioneer in Maternal–Child Advocacy

(February 16, 1881–May 16, 1965)

Mary's Story

Mary Breckinridge came from a distinguished Kentucky family. Her grandfather was a Vice President of the United States under President Buchanan and Secretary of War of the Confederacy under Jefferson Davis. Her father, a career diplomat, was the American Minister to Russia in the Cleveland administration. She was the second of four children and spent four years as a teenager in Russia and Switzerland where she learned French and German. Breckinridge always considered her academic education lacking because of her limited knowledge of mathematics. Her first exposure to nursing was the birth of her brother in Russia when she was 14. Her mother had a family doctor, an obstetrician, and a midwife. Because it was a normal birth, the midwife performed the delivery while both doctors watched (Wilkie & Moseley, 1969; Breckinridge, 1952).

Breckinridge loved to travel and was an avid horsewoman and hunter. Her family's wealth ensured her financial security, but she wanted independence. After a brief marriage, her husband died in 1906. An invitation to visit a girls' school in the mountains of North Carolina led her to her future career. Breckinridge sat with a child with typhoid fever during that trip and realized how helpless she was to care for him. A conversation with Dr. William Polk in New York City led to a letter of introduction to the nursing school director at St. Luke's Hospital and her enrollment. The three years were arduous, but Breckinridge was stubborn and achievement-oriented (Wilkie & Moseley, 1969). Her fear of mathematics wasn't an obstacle because she was tutored by a classmate and a friendly chemist (pharmacist) helped her with each drug problem (Breckinridge, 1952).

Breckinridge's love of children manifested itself during her training when she attempted to adopt an unwanted infant girl with spina bifida, whom she named Margaret. She obtained a doctor's permission and attempted to take the baby from her clinical site, the Lying-In Hospital, to her home site of St. Luke's. Breckinridge, her friend, and the doctor were all suspended on charges of infant abduction. When they explained to a special board, the suspensions were lifted, but Margaret was returned to the Lying-In Hospital, where she died two days later. Breckinridge buried the infant at her own expense and mourned her loss (Wilkie & Moseley, 1969).

After graduation in 1910, Breckinridge went to her parents' home to help her mother, who was in poor health, and didn't practice nursing for several years. She married a professor at a small southern college and delivered her son, Breckie, in August 1914. Breckinridge's life revolved around her family, especially Breckie, and she was ecstatic when she became pregnant again in 1916. Her daughter, Polly, lived only a few hours, but her friendship with her children's French Swiss nurse, Juliette Carni, lasted for many years. On January 23, 1918, Breckinridge's life drastically changed again. After a short illness, Breckie died suddenly. His mother was devastated and her marriage ended in divorce several months later. Eventually, she went to court and resumed her maiden name (Wilkie & Moseley, 1969).

Now, Breckinridge decided to devote her life to service and wrote in her journal: "There is a work beside which all other strikes me as puerile— the work which seeks to raise the status of childhood everywhere, so that finally all of the little ones come into the health which is their due" (Wilkie & Moseley, 1969, p. 37). She wanted to serve in France and enrolled in the American Red Cross Nursing Service. She was assigned to travel the United States for the Children's Bureau to report on the condition of the nation's children and make speeches on their behalf. In 1918, Breckinridge went to Washington to make her final report and found herself in the midst of the influenza epidemic. She volunteered to help and was assigned as assistant to the nurse in charge of one of the four medical areas of the city. Her head nurse became ill and Breckinridge replaced her, caring for about 40,000 patients with five nurses. She labored day and night and her talent for organization blossomed. She organized hundreds of aides—from young government employees to elderly physicians. They did house-to-house visits in slums to care for sick residents. When the epidemic ended, the Armistice was signed on November 11, 1918. The Red Cross no longer sent nurses to Europe, but Breckinridge was determined to go anyway (Wilkie & Moseley, 1969).

When Breckinridge found it would take a few days to get her passport, she went to the Boston Instructive District Nursing Association for special public health and visiting nurse training in preparation for France. Then, she was accepted as a volunteer with CARD (American Committee for Devastated France). After reporting to the Commissioner in Paris, Breckinridge was assigned to Vic-sur-Aisne. The CARD members were all inexperienced volunteers who worked collaboratively to help needy French families. CARD was well organized and women volunteers wore a uniform blue military jacket and skirt to identify them easily. The organization also had chauffeurs for support, an idea that Mary adapted later for the Frontier Nursing Service's couriers (Breckinridge, 1952).

The volunteers began by supplying food, clothes, supplies, and seeds for the people of the Vic. Breckinridge knew that she had to feed mothers so they could nurse their babies and started a program for children under six and pregnant and nursing mothers. She obtained malted milk and chocolate for nursing mothers and started a goat fund to provide milk for children. Her wide circle of influential friends contributed and goats arrived by shipments along with beetroots to feed them. The American ambassador also gave money to buy a buck for breeding. Breckinridge and her colleagues succeeded in preventing starvation. Other organizations partnered with CARD by supplying female dentists and money for extra hot noon meals for children. In 1919, Breckinridge's work extended to the rest of the sector and care for all age groups. In this expanded role, she met with influential nurse leaders and learned that French midwives were well-trained, but not their hospital nurses. She also learned that all English nurses were midwives (Wilkie & Moseley, 1969; Breckinridge, 1952).

Breckinridge returned from France in 1921 convinced that nurse–midwifery would best meet the needs of American children from before birth to age six. CARD also prepared her for beginning the Frontier Nursing Service by its blueprint—start small, become established, and grow by learning about native customs and merging this knowledge with new approaches. CARD taught Breckinridge that facts and data are important and that change must be reality-based. These were lessons she would use throughout the rest of her career (Breckinridge, 1952).

In 1922, Breckinridge entered Teachers College at Columbia University as a non-matriculating student in public health nursing. She enrolled this way because of gaps in her formal education. Breckinridge planned to spend the following summer in rural mountain areas of Kentucky observing conditions there and meeting leading citizens in preparation for her future nursing work. Her time at Columbia was well-spent and she studied social sciences, nursing education, public health, statistics, general and child psychology, and psychiatry (mental hygiene). She also met Dr. Ella Woodyard, who tutored her in decimals and fractions and who would be invaluable to the success of the Frontier Nursing Service (Breckinridge, 1952).

Breckinridge spent the summer of 1923 in the Kentucky mountains. During the course of that summer, she rode 650 miles on 13 horses and 3 mules and talked with 53 midwives. Each midwife's average age was 60.3 years and many were intelligent and clean. Ten were slovenly but at least 16 had more than average ability. The rest were in between. They were superstitious and none had any training for their role. All the midwives Breckinridge spoke with were white, except one. The last two weeks of her journey, Dr. Woodyard came and did mental testing of 66 children from 6–10 years of age. She found that they had a higher average intelligence than the norm for their age group. Dr. Woodyard became fascinated with Breckinridge's vision for nurse–midwifery in Kentucky and later became the research director of the Frontier Nursing Service (Breckinridge, 1952).

The next step in Breckinridge's plan was to go to England and study midwifery herself. In autumn 1923, She sailed to England and met Rosalind Paget, who had founded the Midwives Institute in 1881. Paget was selected as the first Queen's Nurse and was also a Nightingale Nurse. One of Breckinridge's most treasured possessions was a copy of *Introductory Notes on Organizing an Institution for Training Midwives and Midwifery Nurses* by Florence Nightingale, a Christmas gift from Adelaide Nutting at Teachers College. She was honored to meet Paget, who told her to go to the Woolwich in London as a pupil–midwife for a four-month course for trained nurses. Breckinridge enjoyed district nursing there and was required to deliver a minimum of 20 cases of normal births, observe abnormal cases delivered by physicians, attend daily lectures and classes, and pass an oral and written examination to become the first American certificated nurse–midwife. In 1924, Mary Breckinridge became a member of the Midwives Institute (Wilkie & Moseley, 1969; Breckinridge, 1952).

After a few months at home, Breckinridge went to Scotland to see the Highland and Islands Medical Service and met its founder, Sir Leslie MacKenzie. This service included nursing centers and rural hospitals as well as trained nurse–midwives who lived and worked in small outlying communities. The Service was funded as a private enterprise with government support by grants. Voluntary committees in each community provided direct administration. The committees took donations and charged patients small fees. The Crown Grant covered the rest of funding. Nurses were salaried and were provided uniforms and lodging. Nurses shared a cottage for two and had meals served by landladies or assigned maids. They also had complete dispensaries for medications and medical supplies. Fees were based on ability to pay and Breckinridge was impressed with the Service, its administration, and its financial and community support for nurses and clients (Breckinridge, 1952).

After leaving Scotland, Breckinridge returned to the London Post-Certificate School of the Lying-In Hospital as a postgraduate student of midwifery. She took a short introductory course to teach midwifery, worked in antenatal clinics, and delivered babies in the district. She also spent time in Hertfordshire to study services there. This visit gave her ideas for her future endeavor. The county committee there employed a superintendent of nurses who also received a county grant as inspector of midwives. Local authorities, educational leaders, and patients all contributed to fund services, an insurance plan that covered some costs under local administration by voluntary groups (Breckinridge, 1952).

Now, Breckinridge was ready to begin her venture. She chose Kentucky because of its remote rural areas and her belief that success there would lead to success anywhere. She had the advantage of a family name well known in the state and influential friends and relatives. The Health Commissioner gave Breckinridge her certificate to practice in Kentucky and she planned an initial meeting of potential supporters for May 28, 1925, in Frankfort.

The Kentucky Committee for Mothers and Children began at that meeting and launched the first nurse–midwife service in three Kentucky counties. At the time, the death rate for American women in childbirth was the highest in the civilized world. Annually, nearly 20,000 mothers and nearly 200,000 babies died at birth or within one month of delivery. These statistics reflected more maternal deaths than deaths in all wars fought by Americans until that time. The meeting noted the importance of data to determine the effectiveness of the new service. Accomplishments included plans for an annual audit, accurate records, transportation of patients to the nearest city for hospital care, free railroad passes, legal and professional status of nurse–midwives, honorary membership for the state health officer, arrangements for medical consultation, and location of services (Wilkie & Moseley, 1969; Breckinridge, 1952).

After the meeting, Breckinridge began a survey of all births and deaths in Leslie County to determine how many were unreported since registration of births and deaths began in 1911. She obtained forms from the Bureau of Vital Statistics and hired Beetram Ireland from Scotland to do the survey. Ireland was visiting the United States and could ride a horse so she was a logical choice. She surveyed for three weeks and needed additional help. Breckinridge assigned a teacher and the first two nurse–midwives to help complete the survey. They finished the survey in September and found 10% more births and 17% more deaths than reported. This data formed the baseline for the new service (Breckinridge, 1952).

Breckinridge had other activities to occupy her time that summer. She began by underwriting the work for the first three years to meet any deficits, but didn't tell anyone except the treasurer. She obtained a few donations and added $1,000 in the memory of her mother and great-aunt (who she considered her grandmother). Breckinridge opened an account at the Hyden Citizens Bank for payroll and building obligations. Her checks were used as legal tender by citizens and went from person to person with numerous signatures before returning to the bank (Breckinridge, 1952).

With finances out of the way, Breckinridge spent the summer riding through Leslie County. Using the lessons learned from CARD, she enlisted support from leading citizens to form the first branch committee. As she rode from place to place, she cared for sick babies and gave mothers suggestions on feeding and childcare. On August 22, 1925, the first branch committee meeting was held with 35 in attendance. The Service began in a vacant house in Hyden, Kentucky, with no plumbing, but a dispensary, horse barn, and clean well. The two public health nurse–midwives who helped with the survey were soon seeing patients in the surrounding area. The Frontier Nursing Service had begun its work (Breckinridge, 1952).

The Service was incorporated in 1926 and officially became the Frontier Nursing Service in 1928. During those years, Breckinridge and her horse Teddy Bear became a common sight in in the Kentucky hills as she participated in district and clinic care. She also gained more supporters. Since her mother died several years before, her father came to spend his retirement with her. He made minor repairs, groomed horses, and became a beloved member of the Hyden Committee and the community. The mother of one of the nurses came and stayed as unpaid housekeeper. Juliette Carni, Breckie's former nurse, came with her husband and daughter. Juliette became cook–housekeeper with her daughter's help and her husband was in charge of the barn and animals. In addition, groups of women in several states sewed layettes for babies on an ongoing basis (Wilkie & Moseley, 1969).

Breckinridge initially couldn't afford a secretary so she spent many nights with her typewriter ensuring accurate records and report sheets. She diligently kept vouchers for the auditors and gave them accountability for every dollar spent. Later she would use trained statisticians from the Carnegie Corporation to keep records and was able to hire a secretary in December 1925 to help with her busy schedule and correspondence. That was a necessity because Breckinridge spoke at meetings throughout the United States for 6–12 weeks annually to promote the Frontier Nursing Service. Her speeches drew subscriptions and donations although she never asked for money. She believed that people needed to decide whether or not to support the Service without any coercion (Breckinridge, 1952).

Breckinridge bought land on Middle Fork and built Big House, which became Wendover. In December 1925, she dedicated it with a Christmas party for 500 of her neighbors with toys for each child. It served as a hospital as well as her home for three years until Hyden Hospital was built in 1928 (Wilkie & Moseley, 1969). Breckinridge "told the people it [Wendover] was built in memory of [her] children to be used in work for their children" and placed a bronze plaque on the living room chimney that read: "To the glory of God and in memory of Breckie and Polly dedicated Christmas 1925" (Breckinridge, 1952).

Breckinridge also engaged in building nursing outposts at strategic locations. Insurance companies were reluctant to provide fire insurance for Wendover and the outposts because of the remote locations. She met in Louisville with representatives of five companies from New York, Hartford, and Philadelphia to convince them. She assured them that she had extinguishers, spaced buildings properly, used fire-resistant shingles, had a large stone cistern, and would buy a fire hose to provide water in volume. She would install the same system at Hyden Hospital when its 12 beds were built. She also promised never to make nuisance claims. Breckinridge recommended dividing every policy between all five so one didn't run the total risk and told them that they would get a lot of new business in years to come if they took her word. They did and the Service's properties became the best risk these firms had in eastern Kentucky (Breckinridge, 1952).

In January 1929, Breckinridge went to New York City for speaking engagements and surgery at St. Luke's Hospital. While she was there, she heard that Juliette Carni died eight days after childbirth and the baby girl was named Mary after her. She recovered enough to return to Wendover by April, but couldn't ride for hours as in the past (Wilkie & Moseley, 1969). Two young relatives served as messengers for Breckinridge to keep her in touch with activities at the outposts and the Courier Service was born to support the nurses. It was patterned after CARD's chauffeur service in France. The volunteers were girls 19 and older who came as juniors for six weeks to two months during the year. Those who returned were called seniors and stayed as long as they wished. They were responsible for horses' health and for jeeps when they came to the mountains. They also went on calls with the nurses to support them and the families. The committees in the rural communities had able leaders, and donors helped build the six outposts and the Hospital. Support committees were also functioning in major cities to provide funds and materials for the Service (Breckinridge, 1952).

As the Frontier Nursing Service expanded, so did the need for trained nurse–midwives and public health nurses. When she hired a nurse who couldn't ride a horse, Breckinridge gave five riding lessons to every new nurse who needed them. She also hired several nurses who weren't midwives and planned to send them overseas for training on scholarships if warranted by their performance. The Board of Health would license them after course completion. In addition to their nursing roles, they also coordinated building for outposts and learned as they went along (Breckinridge, 1952).

Breckinridge continued to seek money for the budget. The Treasurer set up endowment funds and arranged for a CPA firm to perform audit functions. Cash was difficult to find. The $5 midwifery fee was paid in quilts, chairs, and other household items. The small annual fee for general nursing care was paid in cash or not at all. According to Mary B. Willeford of the Frontier Nursing Service, the average per capita income of 400 remote rural families in 1930–1931 was $85.70. Men either worked on the railroad in the winter or floated logs downriver for sale, a dangerous occupation (Breckinridge, 1952).

In summer 1930, a serious drought impacted the mountain families. Breckinridge surveyed the available food there and took her statistics to Washington to seek help for rural citizens. Her data showed that by harvest time in 1931, 90% of these families would be starving. Her information made a difference and the American Red Cross began providing support in January 1931. Breckinridge asked her supporters for cows and the Frontier Nursing Service gave milk and cod-liver oil to thousands of people before the drought broke in April 1931 (Wilkie & Moseley, 1969).

Breckinridge's niece filmed the nurses' activities year-round and released *The Forgotten Frontier* in 1931 in New York City to portray life in the mountains and keep the Frontier Nursing Service in public view. The film was a financial success and Breckinridge decided to capitalize on it by arranging with International Mercantile Marine to sell tickets for a West Indies cruise in 1931 with the Service receiving 25% of every ticket sold. In late 1931, Breckinridge was riding a new horse named Traveller after the death of Teddy Bear. The horse was nervous and she was wearing her uniform with a cape. As the cape billowed out, Traveller panicked and ran. She had no choice except to fall from the saddle. Breckinridge fractured her second lumbar vertebrae and spent eight weeks in a Bradford Frame followed by a metal brace. She took the cruise wearing a steel brace accompanied by one of her nurses (Breckinridge, 1952).

The Depression impacted the Frontier Nursing Service as well as the rest of the country. Staffing at outposts was reduced from two nurses to one nurse. Administrative cuts occurred and staff nurses took a one-third reduction in pay. Some nurses who could afford it volunteered. Times were lean, but subscribers and supporters stood by the nurses. The majority of nurses stayed and continued to work throughout the 1930s because they believed in their mission (Breckinridge, 1952).

As the Frontier Nursing Service (FNS) expanded, the American Association of Nurse Midwives started in Kentucky in 1928 with all 16 charter members from the FNS. At that time, they were the only nurse–midwives in the United States. Breckinridge was still aware of the importance of data showing the difference made in people's lives by the FNS. Metropolitan Life Insurance Company tabulated each of the first 4,000 maternity cases as each series was completed and their detailed findings had great scientific value. During World War II, Met Life lost many statisticians and the Service did its own tabulation. After the first 1,000 births were tabulated, Dr. Dublin of Met Life stated:

> *The study shows conclusively what has in fact been demonstrated before, that the type of service rendered by the Frontier Nurses safeguards the life of the mother and babe. If such service were available to the women of the country generally, there would be a saving of 10,000 mothers' lives a year in the United States, there would be 30,000 less stillbirths and 30,000 more children alive at the end of the first month of life. This study demonstrated that the first need today is to train a large body of nurse–midwives, competent to carry out the routines which have been established both in the FNS and in other places where good obstetrical care is available. (Breckinridge, 1952, p. 312)*

Met Life also promoted and supported a health insurance plan based on the success of the Frontier Nursing Service where hospital and home care services were available for a yearly fee of $1.00 with the ability to obtain services if patients couldn't pay. This was one of the first managed healthcare groups in the United States (Judd, Sitzman, & Davis, 2012).

The Carnegie Corporation set up the first statistical system for FNS and careful records were kept from prenatal registration to one month post-delivery. The Service accumulated the only large body of OB facts available in the United States on native rural population. More than 99% of mothers were delivered without forceps and few C-Sections were needed. Members of FNS contributed numerous scientific articles of their procedures and results. Since Breckinridge had depended on England and Scotland for postgraduate midwifery training, it was time to develop this training in the United States. The Frontier Graduate School of Midwifery began by training two Native American nurses for a year's postgraduate work in 1935 with FNS. The school officially began in 1939 and the Kentucky Board of Health conducted licensing exams and licensed graduates as certified midwives. The curriculum was based on a six-month course by British schools for graduate nurses, including a minimum of 20 normal deliveries (Breckinridge, 1952).

Breckinridge spent three months in a cast after a spinal fusion in 1938, but continued her work with FNS throughout her life. Her achievements were legendary. Over 1 million dollars of outside money supported the FNS properties. Nurses from within the United States and around the world came to FNS to learn. Breckinridge donated all royalties from her autobiography to FNS and deeded Wendover to it in 1930. When her money ran out in 1938, she took a salary like the workers and Hyden Hospital was renamed Mary Breckinridge Hospital in 1975. The district nursing centers each have a local committee of community members. An Advisory Committee evaluates FNS and informs it of changing community needs and attitudes. Research continues and the FNS participated in the clinical study for the first oral contraceptive. Mary Breckinridge's dream has become a dynamic reality in the Kentucky mountains (Wilkie & Moseley, 1969; Breckinridge, 1952).

The best tribute to Mary Breckinridge came from her organization's first auditor, W. A. Hifner, Jr.:

> *I shall not attempt to describe to you all the beautiful scenes these annual reports have brought to my mind, as they are too many and too varied. Their predominating motif, constantly recurring, seems to be the spirit of an intrepid adventurer and pioneer, wearing a girdle of courage, a mantle of faith and hope, a banner of mercy, and a shield of duty; a spirit imbued with an overwhelming and intense love for little children. (Breckinridge, 1952, pp. 201–202)*

Implications for Nurse Leaders Today and in the Future
Political Savvy

Mary Breckinridge and Florence Nightingale had something in common that today's nurse leaders must emulate. Both were politically savvy and used it to their advantage, Breckinridge in creating and promoting the success of the Frontier Nursing Service and Nightingale in creating the first nurse training school and promoting the success of the nursing profession (Breckinridge, 1952; Cook, 1913a). Their other similarities included a privileged childhood, access to powerful and wealthy allies, and the ability to engage others in all walks of life to support and promote their philosophy and mission (Breckinridge, 1952; Cook, 1913a, 1913b).

Today's nurse leaders must pay close attention to these lessons for their career success and that of their organizations. Leadership and management courses seldom focus on the importance of being politically savvy and developing social intelligence, but both are essential to personal and professional accomplishment. Some nurse leaders, like Breckinridge and Nightingale, have naturally developed these skills, but others can learn to achieve them. According to Rebecca Shambaugh (leadership strategist and founder of Women in Leadership and Learning), there are five ways to develop social intelligence and political savvy (2012).

1. *Situational Awareness:* Read people's emotional states, willingness to interact, and possible intentions and goals. Develop a social aptitude: Network with key stakeholders. Find out about their needs, concerns, and goals.

2. *Presence:* ...to have presence, know and state your opinions firmly, backing them with strong rationale. Don't personalize: See business as business. Feelings don't count. Organizational goals do.

3. *Authenticity:* Being authentic is being honest, open, trustworthy, and with good intentions...you'll also be in a position of strength if you hear others out first and then, based on their concerns, advocate your views. Step back, read the environment, ask people questions, see where they sit on the issue, and then build your case, advocate your views, or state your recommendations.

4. *Empathy/connectedness:* Being attentive to others and adapting your language to your audience, seeing others' points of view, making your point be asking insightful questions, giving the big picture, avoiding irrelevant details, listening attentively, and giving others credit strengthens your position.

5. *Clarity:* Having clarity is being decisive in the way you say things and getting to your point rather than letting others direct you. It's the ability to explain your views in a way that makes others want to join your proposed course of action. You can do this by owning your message and using active voice followed by a strong rationale in a confident statement.

In addition to Shambaugh's five key ways to develop social intelligence and political savvy, it is important for nurse leaders to know that politically savvy individuals also approach situations calling for change in an ethical manner. There is nothing false about political savvy. It is genuine and honest. Although nurse leaders hold formal positions in their organization, much of the effectiveness of social intelligence and political savvy occurs behind the scenes as informal strategies to facilitate change. Politics exist in all organizations and are not inherently good or bad. Savvy leaders are also ethical leaders of high integrity who focus on doing the right thing and what is best for the organization and those it serves (Brandon & Seldman, 2004).

Breckinridge and Nightingale role-modeled social intelligence and political savvy. Today's nurse leaders must develop their own skills in these leadership approaches for their professional advancement and the success of their organizations, with the ultimate goal being attainment of the organization's mission, vision, and values.

— 10 —

Margaret Sanger
Family Planning Activist

(1879–September 14, 1966)

Margaret's Story

Maggie Louisa Higgins was born in Corning, New York, the 6th child in a family of 11 children. As a child, Maggie saw how each succeeding pregnancy caused serious health issues for her mother. Anne Higgins was pregnant 18 times in 30 years of marriage. She contracted tuberculosis shortly after her marriage (Whitelaw, 1994). In spite of her ill-health, Anne always worked and took in washing because her husband, Michael, was ostracized by the neighbors for being a Socialist who criticized the government, laws, the church, and religious traditions. This resulted in an economic boycott of his business as a stonemason (Whitelaw, 1994; Douglas, 1975). Higgins adored her father and admired his views. She always adhered to his philosophy: "Leave the world better because you, my child, have dwelt in it" (Whitelaw, 1994).

Higgins also learned to face her fears and fight for her rights during her youth. She wanted to be a reformer like her father, but tried to avoid situations where she couldn't win. After being scolded by a teacher in eighth grade, she refused to return to the local school. Because the family believed in education for girls, her two older sisters arranged for her to attend Claverack

College, a co-ed school in the Catskills. They guaranteed her expenses and she worked by waiting tables and washing dishes in the school dining room to pay for the rest of her board. There, she became Margaret and took courses in public speaking, painting, and literature. She was a lovely young woman who became friends with other young women who enjoyed arguing and rebelling against authority (Whitelaw, 1994; Douglas, 1975).

At first, Higgins had difficulty with public speaking. She went to a nearby cemetery and rehearsed in front of the graves. She managed to speak on women's rights and starred in several plays during her years at Claverack (Whitelaw, 1994).

After three years, her sisters were unable to continue financing her education and she returned home to care for her mother who was gravely ill. After her mother's death, Higgins kept house for her father and younger siblings. She was 20 and wanted to do something else with her life. She considered becoming a doctor, but couldn't afford the years of study involved. Instead she enrolled in nursing school at White Plains, New York. She received room and board as well as a small salary for hospital work (Whitelaw, 1994).

During her arduous training, Higgins developed tuberculosis herself and later had two glandular surgeries. She continued her studies and did maternity cases in homes during her third year of training. Higgins delivered many babies and began her lifelong love of childbirth. She considered childbirth a divine experience and felt like praying when she held a newborn. Many of these women had multiple births and were in poor health, but didn't know how to prevent future pregnancies. At the time, Higgins didn't know either and was upset by her own inability to help them (Douglas, 1975).

In her final rotation at Manhattan Eye and Ear Hospital, Higgins met an architect who was several years older, named William Sanger, at a dance. It was a whirlwind courtship and Bill arranged an impromptu wedding in the two hours she was off-duty in August 1902. Shortly after, she left nursing school and moved into a Manhattan apartment with Bill. Her tuberculosis returned and Sanger spent weeks in a sanatorium resting prior to the birth of their first child, Stuart, in November 1903. Stuart's birth was a traumatic experience. Sanger had an inexperienced physician and a lengthy, agonizing labor. She spent the next eight months at the sanatorium with her baby and a nurse who lived next door in her cottage there. Finally, a doctor told her to do something with her life to combat her depression. The next day, she returned to New York City with the baby and the nurse (Douglas, 1975).

Bill built a house on Hastings-on-Hudson and Sanger was pregnant with their second child when they moved in. Then, disaster struck. Bill lit a fire in the fireplace and the steam pipes overheated, causing a fire that destroyed the home. No one was hurt and Grant was born shortly afterward. After rebuilding, the family moved back in, but Sanger was unhappy there. According to her, "[she] was not able to express [her] discontent... but after [her] experience as a nurse with fundamentals this quiet withdrawal into the tame domesticity of the pretty riverside settlement seemed to be bordering on stagnation" (Douglas, 1975, p. 21).

After the birth of their third child, Peggy, in 1910, Sanger's life changed again. Peggy contracted polio that left one leg shorter. Sanger still loved nursing and children, but not the work involved in caring for them. She and Bill sold the land and moved to an apartment in New York City where his mother lived with them and did the household and child care tasks. The arrangement was a good one and Sanger began to help with childbirth in the tenements of New York. Daily, she climbed stairs to laboring women past garbage and stale odors to bring a new life into the world. Most of these mothers already had several children and had no resources or strength to care for them as well as the new baby. Women, using unsafe procedures that caused injury and even death in some cases, aborted one of every five pregnancies themselves (Whitelaw, 1994).

Sanger tried to help these women by explaining about withdrawal and condom use. Neither approach was helpful for the poor. Women knew that men used condoms when visiting prostitutes and refused to mention them to their husbands. They didn't have money to buy products themselves or knowledge about them. The other issue was the Comstock Laws that had made mailing information about contraceptive materials illegal forty years before. Some states also had laws restricting publication and circulation of contraceptive information and many doctors believed that women should not be allowed to make decisions about family planning (Whitelaw, 1994).

In 1912, an incident occurred that changed Margaret Sanger's life and the lives of many women in the United States. In mid-July, she and a doctor cared for Sadie Sachs, a woman in her 20s who had performed a self-induced abortion. She wanted to know how to prevent future pregnancies and the doctor laughed and told her to keep away from her husband. In October of that year, she was again called to attend to Sadie, who died of another self-induced abortion. Sanger found her cause. Now, she needed to educate herself before she could help others. She spent time talking with doctors and studying the subject in libraries, but couldn't find information about the needs of normal married people (Douglas, 1975).

The editor of the *Call*, a Socialist paper, asked Sanger to speak to a women's group that year. Her message was that everyone deserved good health. The second meeting drew 75 women to discuss the theme that all children should be wanted. Then, she began writing for the paper about contraceptives. In November 1912, Sanger wrote a series of articles called *What Every Girl Should Know* where she explained about a woman's body and reproductive cycles and cautioned against sexual diseases. Sanger's first confrontation with authority and the Comstock Laws came that month when the Post Office seized that *Call* issue because those laws made it illegal to mail material about sexually transmitted diseases (Whitelaw, 1994).

In October 1913, Bill, Margaret, and the children went to France—he to study painting and she to study France's work on contraception. French wives discussed sex openly and the laws let children share equally in estates. This provided an incentive for men to keep families small by using contraception, though French wives were responsible for limiting household numbers. Smaller families were more prosperous. Sanger learned that abortions were readily available by reputable surgeons. The French dependence on abortion as a solution wasn't the answer for Margaret Sanger and she wanted to return home after studying contraceptive methods. Bill wanted to change careers and become a painter so he elected to stay in France. Margaret Sanger and the children left on New Year's Eve 1913 for New York (Douglas, 1975).

On her return, Sanger decided to publish a monthly newspaper, the *Woman Rebel*, "to stimulate working women to think for themselves and to build up a conscious fighting character" (Whitelaw, 1994, p. 47). She wanted to provide practical advice about contraception and spent three months writing, speaking to groups, and advertising the newspaper. The first copies were sent in March 1914 and, in April, the postmaster labeled the issue "lewd, vile, filthy, and indecent" (Whitelaw, 1994, p. 50). The Post Office refused to mail the issue and subscribers wanted their money back (Whitelaw, 1994).

In August 1914, Sanger was arrested on charges of breaking the obscenity laws with a possible sentence of 45 years. While awaiting trial, she wrote a brochure called *Family Limitation* that became the first handbook on birth control. In it, she said that effective use of contraception would make abortion unnecessary. She had 100,000 copies secretly printed and she and friends wrapped, weighed, and stamped bundles of these pamphlets with the notice "Three hundred thousand mothers...lose their babies every year from poverty and neglect... Are the cries of these women to be stifled?... The women of America answer no!" (Whitelaw, 1994, p. 52).

That fall, Bill returned to care for the children, and Sanger, afraid she wouldn't get a fair trial, decided to leave the country before her trial. In October 1914, she took a train to Canada, obtained a new passport under an alias, and wrote from Montreal to mail the bundles of pamphlets. As she sailed to England, she asked Bill for a divorce because they had grown apart over the years. He refused and she put the matter aside for a time. She made friends in England's birth control movement and studied at the British Museum about the history of family limitation and the dangers of overpopulation (Whitelaw, 1994).

January 1915 was significant for both Margaret and Bill Sanger. She went to Holland to visit the world's first chain of birth control clinics. Dutch women had the lowest death rate from pregnancy in the world and their doctors recommended that women space their children two to three years apart. She enrolled in a class for midwives there and learned how to fit diaphragms. Back home, Bill was arrested for openly distributing *Family Limitation* and was sentenced to 30 days in jail.

Mary Ware Dennett created the first American birth control organization— the National Birth Control League. The League's focus was peaceful change of existing laws. When Margaret Sanger contacted her after her return in early October 1915, she refused any support and rejected Sanger's idea that doctors should place birth control devices to protect women from improper procedures and make birth control more acceptable to the public (Whitelaw, 1994).

Bill's mother died and the children were being cared for by others, including friends and Margaret's sister. After Sanger's return, Peggy contracted pneumonia and died at age five. Sanger took care of her until her death and prepared for her trial. Newspaper articles gained her national support and nine of England's most famous authors sent a letter to President Wilson asking him to use his influence for her. Sanger also had support from New York's top social register and a *Night before the Trial* dinner drew 200 people. Suddenly, Margaret Sanger had the support of the National Birth Control League. After several postponements, the government elected not to prosecute the case and Sanger became a national figure of protest against an unjust law. However, no changes were made to the Comstock Laws (Douglas, 1975).

In the two years since the original indictment, it had become clear that Margaret Sanger was not a "disorderly person" (Douglas, 1975, p. 93) nor a publisher of obscene articles. Birth control was now a serious topic of discussion in the country and Sanger began a lecture tour in April 1916 to promote birth control leagues and clinics. She still rehearsed her speech, this time on the roof, before addressing groups. She spoke all over the country 119 times the first year using one basic speech, "The first right of every child is to be wanted" (Douglas, 1975, p. 95). Some venues refused her entrance and other groups boycotted her speeches, but many locations hosted overflow crowds and her message was spreading (Douglas, 1975).

Stuart and Grant were happy at boarding schools and both remained close to their mother. With their satisfaction ensured, Margaret Sanger was free to concentrate on another edition of *Family Limitation* with Dr. Marie Esqui. The publication would be translated into 13 languages and sell over 10 million copies in coming years. Section 1142 of the New York State Penal Code said that no one could give contraceptive advice for any reason. It did contain an exemption that allowed physicians to prescribe them for curing or preventing disease. Using this as a loophole, Sanger began the process of selecting a clinic site in New York City. She studied vital statistics of each borough, wage scales, and number of social agencies in the area to select a location in Brownsville. Her sister Edith (also a nurse) joined Sanger and Fania Mindell (a supporter who spoke Yiddish) to open the Brownsville Clinic where they would size diaphragms for women and use charts to demonstrate placement, but wouldn't fit them. She also notified the district attorney of the opening, but got no response (Douglas, 1975).

In October 1916, the first birth control clinic outside the Netherlands opened in Brownsville. The two nurses saw 140 women the first day and kept track of vital statistics, including births, deaths, abortions, and miscarriages. They provided information about diaphragm use and told the women where to buy the product. The clinic operated for nine days. Then, a policewoman came posing as a client and came back to arrest them. The police ransacked the place and took 460 records. Margaret Sanger was marched down the street to jail where she spent the night with bedbugs, roaches, and rats. When reform society ladies came the next morning, she told them to "clean up the filthy place" (Douglas, 1975, p. 108).

While free on bail, Margaret Sanger and Ethel began seeing clients again and were arrested again for "maintaining a public nuisance" (Whitelaw, 1994, p. 76). This time they were evicted and all three women were charged: Sanger and Ethel for violating Section 1142 and Fania for selling indecent literature (*What Every Girl Should Know*). Now, they had the support of the Committee of One Hundred, a group of wealthy women founded by Juliet Rublee whose husband was a member of the Federal Trade Commission. This time, Sanger engaged a lawyer, J. J. Goldstein, to test if the state could interfere with a person's right to life and liberty (Whitelaw, 1994).

Ethel was tried first, sentenced to 30 days in the workhouse, and a $250 fine. She began a hunger strike that ended 5 days later when she was tube fed by force. Fania was convicted next and a wealthy supporter paid her $50 fine. A panel of three judges heard Margaret Sanger's case. The District Attorney subpoenaed 30 mothers and asked why they went to the clinic. The reply was "to stop the babies" (Douglas, 1975, p. 119). Goldstein brought out their backgrounds—poverty, ill health, multiple pregnancies and children, and abortions and miscarriages. Their testimony upset one of the judges and he adjourned the court. At the next session, the District Attorney emphasized that Margaret Sanger was not a physician and violated the law by showing instructions for use of a cervical cap. She refused to plead guilty and stated, "I cannot promise to obey a law I do not respect." (Douglas, 1975, p. 122).

Sentenced to 30 days at the Queens County Penitentiary, Sanger was impressed with its cleanliness and matron. She spent the month lecturing inmates on "sex hygiene" (Douglas, 1975, p. 125) and obtaining books for an imprisoned former teacher to teach classes for other inmates. She lost 15 pounds during the month because of poor food and her tuberculosis flared again. A delegation of Brownsville mothers met her upon release and she celebrated her freedom at a breakfast party (Douglas, 1975).

Before the clinic, Sanger collaborated with Frederick Blossom, a social worker, to create a magazine called *Birth Control Review*. The first issue was published while she was in prison. He also found someone to finance a picture, *The Hand that Rocks the Cradle*. The film starred Sanger as herself caring for someone like Sadie Sachs with her trial as the climax. The Commissioner of Licenses suppressed the film. Blossom was unstable and divorced his wealthy wife. When he and Sanger became estranged by their views about World War I, he stripped the office bare, taking furniture, files, records, and funds. Juliet Rublee helped keep the *Review* alive and solvent by incorporation of the New York Women's Publishing Company and its circulation rose to 10,000 (Douglas, 1975).

In 1917, Sanger discovered that the U.S. Army used her section on venereal disease from *What Every Girl Should Know* as education for its soldiers. She was about to win another victory. In January 1918, her conviction was upheld since she was a nurse, not a doctor. The court's interpretation changed the intent of the law when it said that licensed physicians could give contraceptive advice "for the cure and prevention of disease" (Douglas, 1975, p. 135), defined as "any change in the state of the body which caused or threatened pain and sickness" (Douglas, 1975, p. 135). This interpretation changed the law to one that would protect ailing mothers since pregnancy sometimes causes pain and sickness. Sanger's strategy paid off.

Later in 1918, Sanger needed a rest so she and Grant spent three months in Coronado, California. Stuart was preparing to enter Yale so he couldn't join them. While there, she worked on a book *Woman and the New Race*, where she stated that famine, war, and poverty were caused by overpopulation and advocated repeal of the Comstock Laws to lower the birth rate and reduce the number of workers competing for jobs. The book was published in 1920 and sold over 200,000 copies (Whitelaw, 1994).

In 1920, Sanger returned to London and Europe and renewed friendships there. Author H. G. Wells had the following to say about her: "When the history of our civilization is written, it will be a biological history, and Margaret Sanger will be its heroine" (Whitelaw, 1994, p. 90). However, France and Germany had banned contraception and were giving bonuses for women to produce children to replace those lost in the War. She was ill throughout the trip and had a tonsillectomy in London for a recurrence of the tuberculosis (Whitelaw, 1994).

In 1920, Margaret Sanger finally obtained a divorce from Bill. There was a new man in her life who would lend his support and money to her cause (Douglas, 1975). His name was J. Noah Slee, a semi-retired executive of the Three-in-One Oil Company. They were polar opposites: she was 42, he was 60; she was an atheist, he was a former Sunday school superintendent; she was Socialist, he was Republican; she was always struggling with finances, he was a millionaire. Noah's personal and financial backing gave Sanger opportunities to spread her message that would otherwise have been challenging (Whitelaw, 1994).

In 1921, Sanger's chief project was the first National Birth Control Conference in New York. The National Birth Control League had dissolved. She used the Conference to launch the American Birth Control League and purposely scheduled it for the same dates as the American Public Health Conference. That way, some of the public health delegates could attend her various sessions. The physicians' session drew 1,000 doctors and she instructed physicians in techniques and current methods of contraception (Douglas, 1975).

The conference was a historic milestone in the birth control journey and even a problem at the final evening rally worked to Sanger's advantage: The town hall site was locked by order of the Archbishop. Sanger was arrested with a supporter when she attempted to speak and was released the next morning. The incident made the *New York Times*, the *Tribune*, and the *Saturday Evening Post*, giving Sanger publicity about free speech, free assembly, and democratic government. When the cases were dismissed the following day, the meeting was rescheduled for the next week at the Park Theater with twice the seating. It attracted an overflow crowd of 2,000 and a new sponsor, the pastor of St. George's Episcopal Church (Douglas, 1975).

At the Archbishop's request, a police investigation and new hearing dragged on for months without action. Noah and Juliet Rublee were called as witnesses. Since Juliet's husband was a lawyer, the members of the Bar closed ranks to support her. According to the *World* publication, "the score today is all in favor of the birth control advocates, not because of the excellence of their case, but because of the sheer stupidity of the opposition" (Douglas, 1975, p. 162).

Margaret Sanger's fame was spreading. The next year, she was invited to participate in a lecture series in Japan. After the Japanese Consul refused to grant her a visa, she obtained one for China and requested permission to land on arrival in Tokyo. Her ploy worked and she met with Japanese officials and convinced them to accept a permanent birth control committee. After seeing China, she, Noah, and Grant went to Egypt, Venice, Paris, and London. She also agreed to marry Noah as long as she could keep her name and come and go as she pleased. Since divorce was not accepted in American society, they agreed to keep the marriage secret for as long as possible. Noah continued to give thousands of dollars to support her American Birth Control League (Whitelaw, 1994).

Sanger attended the 5th Annual Neo-Malthusian and Birth Control Conference in London and invited its delegations to the United States for their 6th annual meeting in 1925 (Douglas, 1975). Back home, she decided to open another clinic and hire a doctor to prescribe the contraceptives. She also sought private funding to pay fees for women who couldn't pay for services. Dr. Dorothy Bocker agreed to this arrangement and Sanger rented an office on 5th Avenue. Two supporters paid Dr. Bocker's salary for one year and provided office equipment. The new organization, called the Clinical Research Bureau, opened in January 1923 and 2,700 women registered for services by the end of February. Dr. Bocker fitted 900 of them with diaphragms for "health reasons" (Whitelaw, 1994, p. 114). Sanger demanded careful patient records—which would be a rich source of research information—and fired Dr. Bocker when she discovered that her records were not good or reliable. Her next physician, Dr. Hannah Stone, was an excellent statistician. She presented her data at the 1925 International Conference in New York and showed that diaphragm use was 98% effective. The *Medical Journal and Record* reviewed her statistics and discussed birth control for the first time in a professional journal. The birth control movement was becoming socially acceptable (Whitelaw, 1994).

The rest of the decade was a busy time for Margaret Sanger. She continued to travel and speak extensively, planned a successful international conference on population control in Geneva, and wrote a new book (Whitelaw, 1994). When the Harvard Liberal Club invited her to dinner, the Mayor of Boston threatened to revoke the license of any hall if she spoke. Then, the

Club invited her as a silent guest and she stood on stage with her mouth taped while her speech was read to a full house. The subsequent publicity was enormous (Douglas, 1975).

When Sanger returned from Geneva, she was still President of the American Birth Control League. Changes had been made in her absence that made the President accountable to the Board. She found that the organization had money in the bank, but hadn't sent out *Review* subscriptions. This reduced the number of subscriptions from 13,000 to 2,500. When Sanger ordered renewal slips sent immediately, she was told it was a Board decision. The League wanted to preserve the status quo and Sanger's activist philosophy was not welcome. She resigned the presidency and eventually left both the League and the *Review* (Douglas, 1975).

The Clinical Research Bureau continued to grow and the inevitable happened in April 1929. Sanger was caring for Stuart, who was ill, and was at her New York apartment. When she was told that the police had raided the Bureau, she left Stuart with the maid and went to the Bureau. An undercover policewoman had posed as a patient and returned with others to arrest the staff, interview patients, and seize records. It resembled the Brownsville raid, but this time proved different. In addition to calling her lawyer, Sanger called Dr. Robert L. Dickinson, chair of the Committee on Maternal Health of the American Academy of Medicine. This time, many doctors offered to testify for the defense due to concern for doctor–patient privileges and the New York Medical Society passed a resolution condemning the seizure of patient records. The second trial's verdict strengthened birth control clinics everywhere (Douglas, 1975).

Although the old laws were still unchanged, more birth control centers were established in the United States. Approval of birth control, sex education, and legislative changes elicited the approval of the National Council of Jewish Women, General Federation of Women's Clubs, the Presbyterian, Unitarian, Universalist, and Methodist churches, the Central Conference of American Rabbis, and the Federal Council of Churches of Christ. The Clinical Research Bureau expanded thanks to the purchase of a New York mansion by Noah. It kept valuable data about incomes, social, economic, health, and sexual information, as well as the medical progress occurring in methods of contraception (Douglas, 1975).

Illegal abortions increased in the Depression years and Sanger focused on serving the poorest women in the country by enabling nurses and other medical personnel to prescribe contraceptives when women couldn't afford to see a doctor. In 1937, North Carolina began state health clinics to offer birth control services followed by 6 other states. By the end of 1939, there were 539 birth control clinics in 42 states. Sanger's next focus on southwest migrant farm laborers resulted in 25 camps in Arizona and California that offered birth control services. She also sat on a presidential committee on health and welfare where she argued for public funding of birth control (Whitelaw, 1994).

Margaret Sanger became honorary chairman of the Birth Control Federation of America, the forerunner of the Planned Parenthood Federation of America. She urged the organization to sponsor research into cheaper and simpler methods of birth control. From 1942–1943, her major focus was on caring for Noah who had a stroke and died in June 1943. Both her sons were now doctors serving overseas and both came home safe at the end of World War II (Whitelaw, 1994).

In 1946, Sanger went to Europe to help organize family planning conferences in Sweden and England. While she was there, she organized an international birth control committee that became the International Planned Parenthood Federation. In the 1950s, she traveled to Japan, India, and Stockholm to support family planning. The nurse who had been reviled in the early years of the century was now the recipient of multiple awards and honors for her pioneering work in family planning. She was even considered for the Nobel Prize (Whitelaw, 1994).

Margaret Sanger had health problems for several years prior to her death in 1966, but she lived to see development of a safer, more effective birth control pill that was available for general use in 1960. In June 1965, Griswold vs. Connecticut struck down the Comstock Laws based on right to privacy. Margaret Sanger won her battle (Douglas, 1975).

Remembering Michael Higgins's advice to his daughter Maggie, Nancy Whitelaw summed up Margaret Sanger's inspiration in this way: "Millions of us are inspired to fight for what we believe in, to leave the world better because we have dwelt in it" (Whitelaw, 1994, p. 152).

Implications for Nurse Leaders Today and in the Future
Importance of Statistical Analysis

Margaret Sanger and Florence Nightingale both understood the importance of statistical analysis to the success of their endeavors (Douglas, 1975; Cook, 1913a, 1913b). Today's nurse leaders review multiple data sources, research studies, and statistical reports to make clinical and administrative decisions that affect the functioning of the unit, division, and facility. This is a huge responsibility and they must understand the meaning of these datasets and reports before they can develop and implement choices that influence the bottom line and, most of all, quality patient care. Nurse leaders must determine if research results related to nurse-sensitive indicators are statistically or clinically significant and critically analyze the impact of these results on their daily practice. They need to begin by defining the difference between statistical and clinical significance:

> *A statistically significant difference means an association or difference exists between the variables that wasn't caused solely by normal variation or chance. (Heavey, 2015, p. 26)*

> *A difference is deemed clinically significant when experts in the field believe a statistically significant finding is substantial enough to be clinically important and thus should direct the course of patient care. (Heavey, 2015, p. 27)*

When reviewing these results, nurse leaders must see if the probability value (*p* value) is less than the certainty level (*alpha* value). An *alpha* value of 0.05 means that the results will only occur by chance 5% of the time. A *p* value that is less than 0.05 means that results are statistically significant and didn't occur at random. The variables are related based on the researcher's analysis (Heavey, 2015). If the researcher found that a certain patient population with a high fall risk score are more likely to fall than those with a lower fall risk score (*p* 0.02), the results are statistically significant (Heavey, 2015). However, to be clinically significant, the result must be able to detect fall risk across numerous patient populations. If it cannot do this, experts in the specialty will recommend that it is not clinically significant and shouldn't "guide clinical practice" (Heavey, 2015, p. 27).

Nurse leaders must also understand how sample size affects statistical results. A sample that is too small may cause a *type II* error by missing a statistically significant difference. Too large a sample may cause a *type I* error by reporting a difference that is due to chance (Heavey, 2015).

When they are analyzing statistical results, nurse leaders must first look at statistical significance and refer to experts to determine if that difference is clinically significant. Nurse leaders must carefully evaluate statistical results to decide if they should direct clinical practice (Heavey, 2015). Nightingale demonstrated the importance of statistical analysis in "her scheme for Uniform Hospital Statistics" (Cook, 1913a, p. 431). Sanger's Clinical Research Bureau confirmed the need for child spacing and assessed the value of current techniques. This inspired the first studies in birth control and family living (Douglas, 1975). Today's nurse leaders are in good company as they focus on the importance of statistical analysis.

$$\sim 11 \sim$$

Estelle Massey Riddle Osborne
Administrator and Change Agent

(April 3, 1903–December 12, 1981)

Estelle's Story

Estelle Massey was achievement-oriented. She was the 8th of 11 children of a handyman and farmer and a mother who worked as a domestic. Neither of her parents was educated, but they believed in education for their children. Her mother cleaned white homes, but never allowed her daughters to engage in that work. All 11 children achieved at least two years of college. After high school, Massey attended Prairie View State College and graduated as a teacher. She taught school for two years, but wanted to do something different with her life (Mosley, 2004).

When Massey began working as an assistant to her dentist brother in St. Louis, she wanted to become a dentist. He guided her toward nursing and a new training program at a nearby hospital (old City Hospital No. 2). Massey enrolled in the first class of student nurses and wasn't happy in the beginning. After she learned and gained proficiency in nursing procedures, she found that she actually liked nursing (Mosley, 2004).

After graduation in 1923, Massey passed the Missouri State Board Exam with a score of 93.3% and became the first African American nurse to break the color barrier at the hospital by accepting the position of head nurse at one of the largest wards there (Hine, 1989). She stayed three years and was never encouraged to apply for supervisory positions. She realized that she would always have to work there under white supervision and resigned her position. Massey took a position at the St. Louis Municipal Visiting Nurses and found the same prejudice she had struggled under at Homer G. Phillips. She left that agency after six months and moved to Kansas City, Missouri. She was hired as an instructor at the Lincoln School of Nursing there. Convinced she needed more education, Massey took a bank loan and attended three summer sessions at Teachers College at Columbia University (Mosley, 2004).

In 1929, Massey resigned from her position at Lincoln and became the first recipient of the Rosenwald Fellowship for African American graduate nurses. She was talented and ambitious and seized every opportunity for professional development. She continued her studies at Teachers College and obtained her BS in Nursing Education in 1930. In 1931, Massey became the first African American nurse with a master's degree in nursing educa-tion. With that degree, she became the best-educated African American nurse in the United States (Hine, 1989; Mosley, 2004).

Now, Estelle Massey was ready to move to new opportunities in nursing leadership. She briefly became the first part-time African American instructor on the staff of the Harlem Hospital Nursing School. Then, she accepted the position of Educational Director at Freedman's Hospital in Washington, DC (now Howard University), where she served on a team funded by the Rosenwald Foundation studying the health and welfare of African Americans in the South. Massey was becoming the best-known African American in nursing and the Board of Directors at her alma mater, Homer G. Phillips Hospital, asked her to become the first African American Director of Nursing there (Mosley, 2004).

In the mid-1930s, Massey returned to St. Louis to accept her new posi-tion. A colleague described her thusly: "Tall, had a sense of fashion, wore exquisite jewelry, was noted for her hats, and her sense of grooming and dress" (Hine, 1989, p. 121). She was elegant, dignified, and stood out in any crowd. Initially, She married a physician named Riddle, but the marriage did not last, and they subsequently divorced. Since Riddle had no children, she devoted herself to her career and the cause of equality for African American nurses. She had an innate ability to move in and out of integrated and segregated groups easily and developed strong relationships in the Midwest and South that would be advantageous for her as a social change agent (Hine, 1989). As Florence Nightingale developed relationships among multiple constituencies to promote the well-being of soldiers and patients, (Cook, 1913a, 1913b), so would Riddle use her relationships to promote racial equality within the nursing profession.

While at Phillips, Riddle became involved in resurrecting the National Association of Colored Graduate Nurses (NACGN). The organization had been inactive for years, had a dwindling membership, and no clear mission or program. African American nurses considered NACGN irrelevant to their lives and practice. In 1934, NACGN held the first meeting of its Board of Directors and Riddle assumed the presidency of the organization. She delineated the steps to revitalize NACGN by honestly assessing the organization's problems and potential achievements. She also convinced the Board to hire Mabel Keaton Staupers, who would help her reach her goals for NACGN. To gain the support of the nation's African American nurses, Riddle toured the country and spoke with hundreds of them about their concerns. Problems included failing state affiliates, disheartened nurses, and a mostly uninformed public. She decided that she needed to create an information bureau for both African American nurses and the public. She and Staupers publicized NACGN as the recognized organization of African American nurses and she focused on increasing membership (Hine, 1989).

In her five years as President of NACGN, Riddle promoted professionalism, education, and practice opportunities for African American nurses in the United States. Her patient, quiet diplomacy enabled her to negotiate with white nurse leaders and philanthropic backers for support and funding. She actively participated in lengthy, tedious discussions at interracial relations committees and meetings with white nursing leaders and implemented a series of conferences of African American nurses in different regions to strengthen the organization and increase understanding between African American and white nurses. Her commitment to cooperation enabled her to become involved in white nursing organizations as the recognized representative of African American nurses. Riddle knew that African American nurses must understand how their organization was being administered, including openness about financial status. She advocated greater local participation by younger African American graduate nurses and asked other African American nurses to initiate monthly meetings with other African American professional groups. Riddle considered this an opportunity to disseminate information about the worth and work of African American nurses to the community via social workers, teachers, principals, and ministers (Hine, 1989).

She invited white ANA state association secretaries to attend regional NACGN conferences to discuss mutual issues. Few white or integrated hospitals hired African American nurses. Even African American hospitals depended on students and hired few African American nurses. Riddle encouraged African American hospitals to hire African American nurses who could provide economical, reliable, and disciplined skilled care. She also discouraged small southern hospitals from operating nursing schools that reduced the quality of students. She saw nursing as a career for outstanding young women and wanted schools to focus on quality when recruiting nursing students (Hine, 1989).

Riddle's reputation opened more doors for her professionally and for African American nurses. In 1935, she was elected Second Vice President of the National Council of Negro Women, which became the largest group of organized African American women in the United States. The Council considered the development of a viable public health system as one of its chief objectives. The Council and NACGN participated in and supported African American protest campaigns against education and employment discrimination, but Riddle's major objective of integrating African American nurses in the profession was still unfulfilled.

From 1934 to 1944, two NACGN representatives attended the ANA Biennial Conventions to discuss the need for complete integration. In April 1939, Riddle was invited to attend the annual meeting of the ANA Advisory Council in New Orleans. She commented,

> *I have been specially invited to the Advisory Committee meeting of the ANA, which is quite a gain in our striving for recognition from them. The National Organization for Public Health Nursing has been far more liberal than the ANA. This is our first time the latter organization has extended such a courtesy to our organization. I regret so much that Jim Crow is about to spoil it. (Hine, 1989, p. 130)*

Her comments were warranted. African Americans were not welcome at the hotel and she was told to use the freight or service elevator. When Riddle asked the ANA President to protest, she offered to meet Riddle "at the train and enter the hotel's service entrance and elevator" (Hine, 1989, p. 130) and asked her to understand that "neither she personally, nor the ANA can deal with the racial question involved" (Hine, 1989, p. 130). The National League for Nursing Education (forerunner of the National League for Nursing) did not respond and Riddle was encouraged not to attend by the NACGN and her friends. Neither ANA nor NLNE took any action (Hine, 1989).

In spite of such setbacks, Riddle continued to press for social change. Her personal power as an individual and professional African American woman continued to increase. In 1941, few nursing schools were open to African American students. In 1943, she was hired as a consultant to the National Nursing Council for War Service. As the first African American appointee, Riddle was responsible for working with politicians and professional organizations to eliminate discrimination in white schools of nursing and the Armed Services (Mosley, 2004). When the Bolton Bill established the U.S. Cadet Nurse Corps under the United States Public Health Service, Riddle reported significant improvement in educational opportunities for African American women interested in nursing. She also mobilized African American nurses and other groups to ensure inclusion of an antidiscrimination clause in the bill. In her own words,

> *pressure upon the over-all nursing supply helped to reduce racial barriers within the employment and educational areas of nursing. Hospitals and public health agencies which lost large numbers of their nurses to the Army and Navy Corps found it expedient to meet their needs with Negro nurses, although many of them had not previously employed this group. (Hine, 1989, p. 153)*

After two years, the number of nursing schools admitting African Americans went from 18 to 28, the Cadet Nurse Corps enlisted 2,000 African American students and provided money for their education, and the Army and Navy lifted bans on African American nurses (Mosley, 2004).

After the war, Riddle concentrated on improving access to higher education for African American nurses. In 1945, she became the first African American nurse to join the NYU faculty and spent eight years there mentoring African American students and nurses. She also focused on integrating professional organizations. In 1946, she married Herman Osborne and continued to provide leadership for improving race relations within the profession and the country by establishing relationships within professional organizations (Hine, 1989; Mosley, 2004).

In 1948, the ANA House of Delegates integrated the organization and granted individual membership to African American nurses as well as adopting a resolution to establish biracial committees in districts and state associations to implement educational programs that promoted development of intergroup relations. Estelle Osborne was also the first African American nurse elected to the ANA Board of Directors (Hine, 1989). She served until 1952 and, when NLN was created in 1954, Osborne became the Associate General Director and Director of Services to State Leagues for the next 12 years. She had successfully conquered racial prejudices in the nursing profession (Mosley, 2004)

Any discussion of Estelle Massey Riddle Osborne's life would be incomplete without mention of one of her greatest achievements—the inauguration of the Mary Eliza Mahoney Award in 1936 by the NACGN at her urging. The Award recognized outstanding achievement in "nursing and human service" (Hine, 1989, p. 126). When the NACGN merged with the American Nurses Association, ANA continued to issue the award to "African-American nurses who have demonstrated excellence in their field" (Darraj, 2005, p. 114). The 1946 Mary Eliza Mahoney Award recipient went to an administrator, advocate for racial equality in nursing, and social change agent—Estelle Massey Riddle Osborne.

Implications for Nurse Leaders Today and in the Future
Change Agent

Today's nurse leaders must emulate the examples of Estelle Osborne and Florence Nightingale to become successful change agents. Both were shrewd negotiators who attracted others to their causes. In the end, both shaped change within the nursing profession—Osborne by the inclusion of African American nurses in professional organizations and Nightingale by the inclusion of trained nurses in professional nursing (Mosley, 2004; Cook, 1913a, 1913b).

Change in health care is constant and nurse leaders cannot be passive recipients when changes occur. They must lead change in their organizations by being willing to try new approaches and keep pace with best practices. They also are committed to growth, able to influence their colleagues, and pursue change with knowledge and positive communication skills.

"Change agents help others transform by advocating for openness and improvement" (Scott, 2015, p. 311). They are enthusiastic about the change and build networks to support it. They also have referent power that makes others want to follow them and the courage to challenge existing power bases without being offensive. Their passion is about the change, not themselves and they support others through the process. Nurse leaders who are skilled in using change theory are invaluable to their organizations (Scott, 2015).

Nurse leaders may use different change models, but two common ones are Kotter's 8-Step Model and Bevan's Seven Change Factors. Each of these models contains steps for successful change similar to those used by Osborne and Nightingale.

Kotter's 8-Step Model consists of (Scott, 2015):

1. Creating a sense of urgency where there is open discussion about the need to change;
2. Forming a powerful coalition of supporters for change;
3. Creating a vision for change;
4. Reinforcing the vision and communicating it;
5. Removing barriers and obstacles;
6. Creating short-term wins;
7. Focusing on continuous improvement to build on the change; and
8. Maintaining the change in the organization.

Brevan's Seven Change Factors focus on the dynamics of the change process. They provide data about activities the change agent must perform to ensure success. These factors include (Scott, 2015):

1. *Clarity*—clearly explain the purpose of the change and the methods required to implement it;
2. *Engagement*—develop commitment by involving the people impacted by the change;
3. *Resources*—identify and provide essential resources for success;
4. *Alignment*—evaluate all areas impacted to ensure they support the changed behavior;

5. *Leadership*—provide every change agent and leader with the skills and abilities to activate the change;
6. *Communication*—ensure two-way communication to clarify issues, answer questions, and counter all challenges; and
7. *Tracking*—measure and monitor results to confirm that goals are achieved.

These are just two examples of change processes. It is also important to avoid rigidity and remember that flexibility will be needed to deal with uncertainty as the process seeks projected outcomes. Both Osborne and Nightingale were self-motivated and committed to change. Today's nurse leaders should adopt these traits and realize that "change leadership is about creating a vision and fostering major organizational transformation" (Scott, 2015, p. 315). It is also an essential role for leaders in today's rapidly changing healthcare environment.

$$- 12 -$$

Mabel Keaton Staupers

Organizer and Negotiator

(February 27, 1890–November 29, 1989)

Mabel's Story

Mabel Doyle was born in Barbados, West Indies, and arrived in New York City 13 years later with her seamstress mother. Her dentist father followed a year later and she became a naturalized U.S. citizen in 1917. Doyle repeated the sixth and seventh grades at 13 and graduated from the Bronx's P.S. 119 in 1914. She immediately entered Freedman's Hospital School of Nursing (now Howard University) in Washington, DC, and graduated with honors 3 years later. Doyle wanted more independence and an opportunity to serve the community, so her nursing career began as a private duty nurse. In 1918, She married James Max Keaton, a physician, and moved to Asheville, North Carolina. Two years later, they divorced and she returned to Harlem (Hine, 2004).

Mabel Keaton joined two physicians and opened the first African American–owned and managed healthcare facility in Harlem, the Booker T. Washington Sanitarium. She demonstrated passion and proficiency in community organizing, healthcare advocacy, and nursing administration. After a year, Keaton moved to Philadelphia to become Superintendent of Nurses at Mudget Hospital. She worked with officials of the Pennsylvania

State Board on a project to standardize nurses training and spent a few months as resident nurse at Philadelphia's House of St. Michael and All Angels for Crippled Children (Hine, 1989).

Later in 1921, Keaton accepted a fellowship from the Henry Phipps Institute to study tuberculosis social work. When she completed a course at the Pennsylvania School for Health and Social Work, this additional education opened new doors for her: She was offered a position as a medical social worker in Philadelphia's Jefferson Hospital Medical College and in 1922, there was an opening at New York's Tuberculosis and Health Association (Hine, 2004). She assisted with a survey of health needs in Harlem and evaluated the services available to African Americans in city and state TB facilities. Her work attracted attention and praise. This survey was the rationale to establish the Harlem Committee of the New York Tuberculosis and Health Association and Keaton became its first Executive Secretary. This visible position facilitated interaction and relationships with African American political and social leaders in New York City. She held this position for the next 12 years and her primary headquarters and professional contacts were in the northeast (Hine, 1989).

Keaton became known for her organizational skills, humor, and boundless energy as she tackled tuberculosis-related issues (Hine, 1989). She organized health education lectures for the public, established fresh-air summer camps for children, and developed health services that included free exams and dental care for schoolchildren. She also created prenatal clinics and advocated the appointment of African American physicians to TB clinics and hospitals in New York City. In addition to these numerous projects, she remarried in 1931 to Fritz Staupers of Barbados. Since they had no children, Staupers continued her healthcare endeavors. A new opportunity would soon make her a national figure in the fight for equality and integration in nursing across the United States (Hine, 2004).

Staupers became friends with another African American nurse leader named Estelle Massey Riddle and her support made Staupers the first salaried Executive Secretary of the National Association of Colored Graduate Nurses (NACGN) in 1934. With funding from the Rockefeller Foundation and Julius Rosenwald Fund, the group's headquarters were established in New York's Rockefeller Center (Hine, 2004). NACGN was a small organization with a limited number of members, many of whom were apathetic about its future. Mabel Staupers was dynamic and dedicated to "interpreting the Negro nurse" (Hine, 1989) to the American public and eliciting support for equal education, nondiscriminatory employment opportunities, and professional integration of African American nurses. She became a visible presence promoting these issues through NACGN. Lillian Harvey, former Dean at Tuskegee, described Staupers as an individual who was "very interested in young nurses" (Hine, 1989, p. 121) and who "wasn't afraid of anything or anyone in the world...could say whether she thought something was good, bad, or indifferent, worth something or worth nothing and say it in a kind of way with a little tinge of humor that you would not take offense" (Hine, 1989, p. 121).

Staupers was a tireless worker for any cause she believed in and elimination of racial discrimination and full integration for African American nurses was that cause. She and Riddle both traveled countless miles meeting with African American nurses to promote membership in NACGN. She disclosed all organization financial information to present an honest picture to members, saying, "we are telling nurses everywhere how the money is spent and how it is raised" (Hine, 1989, p. 125). Her honesty endeared her to African American nurses considering whether or not to join NACGN. Staupers's leadership helped African American nurses with coalition building, first with local African American leaders of non-nursing organizations like the NAACP and National Urban League. Then, she encouraged organizing interracial citizens' committees and started the first one herself in New York City in 1935, the New York Citizens' Committee. By 1942, there were 12 groups across the United States with the purpose of improving the image of African American nurses and obtaining greater employment opportunities in local hospitals and visiting nurse services. In her own words, "in doing this we are following the trend in other nursing organizations. This is valuable, since the nurse needs help and the layman needs to understand the nurse" (Hine, 1989, p. 126).

Staupers personally built permanent bonds with officers of several national African American–rights organizations and the NACGN. She was expert at generating publicity for African American nurses and persuaded editors of several publications to publish full-length articles about African American nurses, their struggles for equality, and their contributions to African American healthcare delivery. Aware of the importance of favorable press, Staupers worked to improve the quality the *National News*, NACGN's own official publication. For a brief period, it was the chief method of communication with members as its quality improved. In 1942, NACGN's Bulletin

Committee recommended biannual publication and replaced it with a more economical monthly membership newsletter (Hine, 1989).

Staupers used the model of the National Organization for Public Health Nursing (NOPHN) to establish a National Advisory Council for NACGN to expand community and professional contacts in New York City by choosing members who were renowned in their fields to promote integration of African American nurses. She also devoted time to resolve problems of racial discrimination brought to her by African American students and graduate nurses. Since NACGN had limited legal and financial resources, Staupers relied on behind-the-scenes negotiation to attain change and improvement in opening educational avenues for African American students. She urged African American nursing students to apply to the finest nursing schools. When a qualified African American applicant was rejected by Yale and Case Western, Staupers communicated with influential people associated with both schools. She purposely avoided publicity and wrote that "our policy here has been not to embarrass our friends; that is why there has not been a great deal of publicity about much of our work in proportion to the publicity received by other organizations" (Hine, 1989, p. 148). Her efforts paid off when Case Western began accepting African American students in mid-1945 (Hine, 1989).

According to Darlene Clark Hine, "it is a supreme irony that nursing's future is so often connected to war" (Hine, 1989, p. 162). World War II was a turning point for racial integration of African American nurses as the Crimean War was a turning point for British female nurses in war zones. Each of these changes were largely due to a single nurse—Mabel Staupers and Florence Nightingale—and both faced opposition and prejudice in achieving their goals (Hine, 1989; Cook, 1913a).

At the beginning of World War II, the Army and Navy Nurse Corps were segregated and Staupers was determined to integrate African American nurses into both. She created a NACGN National Defense Committee whose members represented African American nurses throughout the country. It was a brilliant political move. In October 1940, she went to Washington to discuss concerns about possible rejection of African American nurses for the Army Nurse Corps with Major Julia Flikke. When definitive action didn't occur as a result of that meeting, Staupers called the leaders of the NACGN National Defense Committee to meet with the surgeon general of the Army and his top aides. The meeting didn't go well. He was adamant about only using African American personnel if separate African American wards were designated in hospitals and where the number of African American troops justified separate facilities—a quota system. He believed that segregation was nondiscriminatory if equal accommodations existed and rejected Staupers's proposal that NACGN accept responsibility for recruiting African American nurses for the Army Nurse Corps as needed. He only agreed to permit the NACGN to assist the American Red Cross. After the meeting, Staupers expressed her opinion: "My position is that, as long as either one of the Services reject Negro nurses, they are discriminated against and as long as either Service continues to assign them to duty as separated units, they are segregated" (Hine, 1989, p. 166).

She set out to challenge the War Department with all resources at her disposal, an arduous task, but one that would change the future of African American nurses. Staupers made her case to President Franklin Roosevelt, who assured fair treatment and nondiscrimination for African American nurses. The president's support did not extend to the War Department, which reflected the surgeon general's viewpoint. She confronted the issue: "We fail to understand how America can say to the world that in this country we are ready to defend democracy when its Army and Navy are committed to a policy of discrimination" (Hine, 1989, p. 168).

When there was no response, she sent press releases criticizing the quotas for joining the Armed Forces Nurse Corps and guided the NACGN National Defense Committee to organize anti-quota protests in local communities. Staupers was aware that the support of white nurses and white society would be essential for her cause. NACGN sponsored regional institutes for key nursing leaders—regardless of race—to discuss plans for action and strategies to mobilize public support. She contacted white nursing groups and publicized the contributions of African American nurses nationally. Staupers advocated coverage of African American nurses inducted in the Army Nurse Corps and used every opportunity to tell their story and gain community support. Since one avenue open to African American nurses was joining the American Red Cross, she promoted enrollment by African American nurses. Even white nurses were disturbed by Army Nurse Corps requirements: Army nurses had to be members of a professional nursing organization, between the ages of 18–35, and unmarried. They received a rank, but less pay and power than men of equal rank (Hine, 1989).

Staupers's campaign was gaining support from the African American press, white philanthropists, and sympathetic white nurse leaders. She also won the hearts and minds of the African American public. When President Roosevelt created a subcommittee on Negro Health under the Federal Security Office of Defense, Health, and Welfare, she was the only female member appointed with her African American male colleagues. Members of this group met with the surgeon general again in March 1941. Again, he refused to reconsider quotas for the Armed Services Nurse Corps. Staupers's response was "since Negro nurses recognize that service to their country [is] a responsibility of citizenship, they [will] fight with every resource at their command against any limitations on their services, whether a quota, segregation, or discrimination" (Hine, 1989, p. 174).

By July 1942, the Army Nurse Corps had accepted 60 African American nurses. Progress was slow, but new legislation in 1943 would provide invaluable assistance to Staupers and the NACGN. Francis Payne Bolton introduced legislation to create the Cadet Nurse Corps and NACGN supported an amendment to ensure that African American student nurses could join the Corps. Mabel Staupers was instrumental in publicizing this opportunity throughout the African American nursing profession. African American nursing programs obtained grants to pay for tuition, fees, and uniforms. Students received $15–$30/month and special uniforms in return for agreeing to serve at least six months after the war ended. Some white nursing schools also accepted African American applicants. By 1945, over 2,000 African American nursing students participated in the Cadet Nurse Corps (Hine, 1989, 2004).

The Bolton Bill helped, but Staupers's crusade was not over. The Navy Nurse Corps refused to induct African American women nurses and the Army assigned African American nurses to care only for German POWs. In 1943, Staupers decided to present her case to Eleanor Roosevelt by sending her letters from African American nurses serving at segregated posts prior to scheduling a meeting with her. Mrs. Roosevelt responded positively and their meeting was amicable. Since 1944 was an election year, Staupers implied that she would go public after the election about African American nurses' dissatisfaction with the Armed Services. Mrs. Roosevelt applied pressure to the new surgeon general of the Army, the secretary of war, and the rear admiral of the Navy to recruit African American nurses. Progress continued to be made slowly. In January 1945, the surgeon general spoke with 300 nurses, politicians, and citizens and mentioned the possibility of a draft to meet nursing needs in the Armed Services. Staupers was outraged and asked him, "If nurses are needed so desperately, why isn't the Army using colored nurses? Of 9,000 registered Negro nurses the Army has taken 247, the Navy takes none" (Hine, 1989, p. 179). Her words caused a firestorm that reverberated across the United States. Their exchange made national coverage and her words were published in almost every African American newspaper in the country. Immediately after, President Roosevelt announced his support for amending the Selective Service Act of 1940 to provide for induction of nurses in the Army (Hine, 1989).

Realizing that fiery rhetoric wasn't enough to win her battle, Staupers marshaled her forces by asking African American nurses to rally in support of NACGN. At the same time, she channeled public anger and sympathy by recommending telegrams to the President that protested the exclusion, discrimination, and segregation of African American nurses. She received national support opposing a draft when large numbers of African American nurses were excluded from service. This time Staupers's efforts paid off and the Executive Secretary of the National Nursing Council for War and the NACGN issued a joint statement that the admission of African American nurses in the Navy would have positive effects (Hine, 1989).

On January 20, 1945, the War Department issued an end to quotas and the Navy Nurse Corps opened its ranks to African American female nurses. Staupers's tireless advocacy and years of labor resulted in the elimination of racial quotas and discrimination by the military and opened doors to service for African American nurses. She also aligned multiple groups into cohesive coalitions to change laws and minds. It was an awesome achievement for a dynamic nurse leader (Hine, 2004).

Mabel Staupers resigned as Executive Secretary of NACGN in 1946 and took a well-earned rest for a while. She had won a great victory and changed the future of African American nurses, but she wasn't finished yet. As early as 1934, she began her campaign for integration of African American nurses in ANA. They could be members of the National Organization for Public Health Nurses (NOPHN), but were barred from membership in any other national professional organizations. In ANA, members had to belong to state organizations to be national members. This membership was denied African American nurses so they were excluded from the national organization (Hine, 1989).

From 1934 to 1944, she and Riddle attended the ANA House of Delegates meetings to press for full integration. They gained many friends, but not their primary objective. In 1944, Staupers advised African American nurses at the four regional NACGN conferences to recommend to their Board of Directors to be "ready and willing to vote for complete integration, if and when the American Nurses Association House of Delegates accept us to full membership" (Hine, 1989, p. 183). In 1948, she got her wish and the ANA House of Delegates accepted African American nurses as individual members. Staupers was ecstatic: "The doors have been opened and the black nurses have been given a seat in the top councils. We are now a part of the great organization of nurses, the American Nurses' Association" (Hine, 2004, p. 612).

After integration within ANA, Mabel Staupers had one more duty to perform. She returned to NACGN as president and persuaded its board to pursue complete dissolution of the organization. It had served its purpose and she guided it to its closure on January 26, 1951. Mabel Keaton Staupers had achieved outcomes that others considered impossible by knowing when to negotiate and when to apply public pressure. Her energy and forward momentum swept African American nurses to racial equality and acceptance (Hine, 1989).

In 1951, the Spingarn Committee of the NAACP selected Mabel for the prestigious Spingarn Medal. Their tribute to her was heartfelt: "You were willing to sacrifice organization to ideals when you advocated and succeeded in realizing full integration of Negro nurses into the organized ranks of the nursing profession of this country" (Hine, 1989, p. 186). It was well-deserved recognition for a truly dynamic nurse leader and activist.

Implications for Nurse Leaders Today and in the Future
Dealing with Difficult People

Nightingale and Staupers had very different approaches to dealing with difficult people, but each was successful. Nightingale preferred to go quietly about her duties in the Crimea, gaining allies in the military and medical professions with her serene demeanor and quality of work (Cook, 1913a). Staupers had a more aggressive approach coupled with the ability to enlist a broad base of support (Hine, 1989). Today's nurse leaders also deal with difficult people when negotiating issues important to them. As Staupers and Nightingale discovered, different approaches must be adapted in challenging situations. Nurse leaders must begin by under-standing the personality types of difficult people they must influence to succeed (Sherman, 2014, p. 61–62):

1. The Volcano is "abrupt, intimidating, arrogant, and prone to making personal attacks";
2. The Sniper is "highly skilled in passive-aggressive behavior";
3. The Chronic Complainer is "whiny, finds fault in every situation, and accuses and blames others for problems"; and
4. The Clam is "disengaged and unresponsive, closing down when you try to have a conversation."

Since the nurse leader cannot easily change others' behavior, she or he must focus on changing self-behavior. This is the most effective strategy because the difficult person must learn different ways of interacting with the leader. There are several effective strategies to use when dealing with these personality types (Sherman, 2014, p. 62):

1. "Don't try to change the difficult person."
   They are accountable for their behavioral change, not you.
2. "Don't take it personally."
   Their behaviors reflect what is happening to them, not anything you have done or said.
3. "Set boundaries."
   Expect to be treated respectfully and don't accept public shouting matches.
4. "Acknowledge the person's feelings."
   It is all right to say 'You seem angry.' It is essential to move chronic complainers to problem solving.
5. "Try empathy."
   This is helpful in deescalating a volatile situation. Sometimes these people just want someone to listen and lack suitable communication skills.
6. "Hold your ground."
   Teach them how to treat you by avoiding challenges. If the person is a Sniper, the nurse leader may have to expose their behavior to others.
7. "Use fewer words."
   Brief messages may be more effective in getting to the goal. Setting a time limit for discussion is also helpful. It is important to focus only on the person's behavior, not on the person.

If the person is in a position of power, negotiating and addressing conflict may be risky, but essential for change to occur. Conflict avoidance can result in nothing being resolved. In these situations, a direct approach is best. The person may be unaware of concerns or the impact of their actions. The nurse leader has a duty to express these concerns for their own sake and the sake of the leader's personal integrity. Avoidance can lead to passivity, discouragement, and cynicism. A private location is best for discussion and support from a human resources representative or employee assistance counselor may be required in emotionally charged situations. Professionalism and respect are important in such discussions. Concerns must be stated clearly and the nurse leader should carefully listen to the response without argument. It is imperative to stay calm, be objective, and clearly state the actions needed (Bowers & Ferron, 2014). At one point, Staupers lost her temper in discussion with the surgeon general and had to change her tactics to achieve the goal of integration for African American nurses in the Army and Navy (Hine, 1989, p. 96). Nightingale exemplified this process in her discussions with physicians and military leaders in the Crimea where she shared her concerns professionally, listened respectfully, and clearly focused on resolution (Cook, 1913a). Today's nurse leaders will find themselves in tough situations where dealing with difficult people is essential to success. Using these approaches will prepare the leader to defuse conflict in dealing with difficult people in work and in life.

Mary Elizabeth Carnegie

Educator and Editor

(April 19, 1916–February 20, 2008)

Elizabeth's Story

M. Elizabeth Lancaster's parents divorced when she was two. She was taken in at three by her maternal aunt and uncle and raised as an only child in Washington, DC. Her two older sisters lived with her mother in Baltimore and she saw them at holidays and family gatherings. She grew up to be well adjusted and flexible. Her aunt valued education and pushed her to succeed. She learned to read at an early age and her cousin taught her to speak French. At four, Lancaster entered kindergarten and did well in the classroom. The next year, the teacher told her aunt that Lancaster was too young to move to first grade. Somehow, her aunt convinced the teacher and school that Lancaster should move forward with her class (Houser & Player, 2007).

She lived with her aunt and uncle for five years until her mother could reunite her family in Baltimore. Elizabeth accepted this change well and spent two years with her mother and sisters. In 1926, Lancaster's mother became ill and could no longer care for the girls. Their aunt came to the rescue again by moving Elizabeth's two older sisters to an apartment in Washington, DC, and taking Lancaster and her mother into her home.

It took a year for her mother's health to improve. After that, her mother remarried and died in 1928, three months after delivering a son (Houser & Player, 2007).

Washington was segregated except for public transportation. She remained unaware of racial prejudice and her childhood was a happy one free from racial concerns (Houser & Player, 2007). Elizabeth attended an all–African American high school until her graduation at 16. She was very religious, sang in the church choir, and played the organ in her Catholic church. She considered becoming a nun, but decided to pursue a professional career instead. Elizabeth wasn't sure what her major should be, but she knew that she had to earn her own way to college. Her first experience with discrimination came when she worked in a local white cafeteria in high school to help her family with expenses. She served fruits and vegetables to white patrons, but was unable to eat there herself.

After high school graduation, she decided to move to New York City where her cousins lived. Her indecision about her future was resolved when a cousin who had attended the Lincoln School for Nurses, an African American nurse training school, recommended it. Lancaster applied and put her age on the application as 18 because the Lincoln School didn't accept anyone under 18. She passed the entrance exam and was accepted. All the instructors and the director were white so there were no African American role models to emulate, but Elizabeth found she loved nursing and the sense of freedom at Lincoln. The patients she cared for in training were Jewish. The hours were long, but she enjoyed her experiences. She loved sports and became active in student affairs, which guided her future direction as a graduate nurse (Houser & Player, 2007).

In 1936, Lancaster's life was forever changed by an unexpected event. The Lincoln School was selected as the site for the National Association of Colored Graduate Nurses (NACGN) convention headquarters. Lancaster served as hostess for student delegates and attended sessions and social events (Schorr & Zimmerman, 1988). She listened to a guest lecturer, Mabel Staupers of NACGN, and learned for the first time about discrimination against African Americans in the country and in the nursing profession. There were few African American role models and no African American nursing history was taught in African American nursing schools. This presentation made Lancaster seek a leadership role in eliminating discrimination after her graduation in 1937. She passed her Boards and accepted a staff nurse position on a medical–surgical unit at Lincoln Hospital, but wanted to work in a Veterans Administration facility. After passing the civil service exam for positions at government hospitals, Lancaster was hired at the VA Hospital in Tuskegee. She had to complete one-year probation there before transferring to the Freedman's Hospital. She now worked solely with African American nurses caring for African American patients and there were no racial concerns (Houser & Player, 2007).

While she was at Tuskegee, she worked nights and volunteered on days for the health department where she supervised untrained midwives. Based on this experience, Lancaster decided that she wanted a bachelor's degree with a major in public health nursing (Schorr & Zimmerman, 1988). After her year of probation was completed, Lancaster transferred to Freedman's Hospital where she worked full-time on nights. While she was there, she took two courses during the day at Howard University. Then, Lancaster got an offer from West Virginia State College, an all-African American school, to work part-time as school nurse and go to school full-time (Houser & Player, 2007). She enrolled there in February 1940. In her role as school nurse, she took night calls and delivered babies because there was no physician in the area. Lancaster graduated in June 1942 with a bachelor's degree in sociology and a minor in psychology (Schorr & Zimmerman, 1988; Houser & Player, 2007).

Her next position in 1942 was as a clinical instructor and supervisor of obstetric nursing at St. Philip Hospital School of Nursing, an African American school at the Medical College of Virginia in Richmond. There were five African American nurses on the faculty and they experienced racial discrimination in the dual system of a school for African American students and a school for white students that was run exclusively by white faculty (Schorr & Zimmerman, 1988). At St. Philip, "all the African American nursing instructors had academic degrees, but not all the white instructors" (Houser & Player, 2007). Nursing instructors typically were called 'Miss' or 'Mrs', but African American nursing instructors were called 'Nurse (last name)'. The African American faculty members taught the African American students to use 'Miss' or 'Mrs', but the issue was not resolved until a new nursing director came in 1943 (Houser & Player, 2007).

Lancaster wanted to join the Navy Nurse Corps, but was denied admission. In the summer of 1943, she attended Teachers College at Columbia University and began a different role in nursing education (Schorr &

Zimmerman, 1988). She acquired a new mentor, Estelle Riddle Osborne, who got Lancaster released from her position at St. Philip's to pursue advanced nursing roles and suggested that Elizabeth accept the position of assistant dean at Hampton University. Elizabeth was to be coached in this role to become dean of a school of nursing. She was also charged with starting the first BSN program in Virginia until a nurse with an MSN could take the position (Houser & Player, 2007). The first students were admitted in February 1944 and, when a white dean was hired, Elizabeth continued as assistant dean and teacher (Schorr & Zimmerman, 1988).

Lancaster decided to pursue a master's degree herself and obtained a fellowship from the Rockefeller Foundation to attend the University of Toronto. She studied nursing school administration that led to a certificate of completion. While in Toronto, Elizabeth also met and married Eric Carnegie. When Elizabeth returned home, their marriage continued as a long-distance relationship for 10 years. They eventually divorced because Eric wouldn't move to the United States and she wouldn't move to Canada (Houser & Player, 2007).

During that decade, Carnegie's career flourished partly due to the Rockefeller Foundation. Florida A&M applied to the Foundation's General Education Board for funding to build a hospital. The Board agreed, on the condition that the A&M School of Nursing be reorganized under the supervision of a nursing dean instead of a hospital medical director. Since Elizabeth Carnegie's Nursing Administration Certificate was equivalent to a master's degree, she had the proper credentials and was accepted as nursing dean. Although A&M's administration accepted Carnegie's degree, she could not consider it equal to a master's degree. After a few years at A&M, Carnegie asked the Rockefeller Foundation for another grant: "You have got to give me another scholarship to complete my master's degree before I can continue in this position at Florida A&M" (Houser & Player, 2007, p. 45).

With her new fellowship, Carnegie attended the Syracuse University Master of Education program. The program focused on higher education and Syracuse accepted her Canadian education credits. She took this route rather than repeating the entire year in the MSN program. Carnegie took an additional nursing course each semester to keep pace with changes in nursing education and returned to her position at A&M after graduation (Houser & Player, 2007).

At that time, Florida A&M had the only BSN program in Florida. However, on Carnegie's arrival in 1945, the students' clinical experience was deficient. Students had to spend an additional year at an affiliated school in Baltimore before they were prepared for the Board exam. In her own words, "I walked into an organizational disaster and had numerous critical issues facing me, all needing attention immediately" (Houser & Player, 2007, p. 46). Her immediate priorities were to reorganize the school, seek national accreditation, and make the school an integral part of Florida A&M. She saw an opportunity to help African American nurses gain the respect of the public and their nursing colleagues (Houser & Player, 2007).

Carnegie found no standard selection criteria for student nurses. There were no records, no high school transcripts, no birth certificates, and no aptitude test scores. She began by administering a national aptitude test that weeded out half the students. Her struggle to raise academic standards was frustrating and she considered quitting her position. The Rockefeller Foundation encouraged her to stay and supported her changes (Houser & Player, 2007).

Carnegie focused on finding different clinical sites for the nursing students. She sought closer affiliations that would provide her students with quality clinical rotations and requested permission to visit larger facilities in Florida. Once permission was granted, she began her search. Most of the facilities had white directors and the prejudice against African Americans was palpable. Directors refused to respond to her handshake and she couldn't place her nursing students in those facilities where they might be mistreated. Finally, she went to the Duval Medical Center in Jacksonville. The white director readily shook her hand and made her feel welcome. She also helped obtain permission for the A&M students to do clinical experiences there (Houser & Player, 2007).

Now, Carnegie had to find funds for student housing in Jacksonville. She convinced the A&M president to request and obtain funds from the Rockefeller Foundation for the students. The Foundation was generous and a house was purchased to house 12–16 nursing students. Funds also paid for faculty members, a cook, a dietitian, office furniture in space set aside by the hospital, a small library of books, and a furnished classroom (Houser & Player, 2007).

The contract was signed, but Carnegie ran into a problem at the Duval Medical Center that was similar to the issue she experienced at the St. Philip Hospital. This time it related to how the African American student nurses should be addressed. White nursing students were called 'Miss', but African American students were called 'Nurse'. Carnegie dealt with this by reminding the director that the African American students couldn't be called 'nurse' because they weren't nurses yet. That resolved the issue and African American nursing students were called 'Miss' the same as their white peers (Houser & Player, 2007).

One week before the first clinical rotation in Jacksonville, another problem arose. According to the Jacksonville paper, white nurses at Duval threatened to walk out if the African American students entered the facility. The A&M students conducted themselves with dignity and the strike never materialized. The first year, the A&M students could only staff wards with all African American patients. Within the year, they were welcomed on all nursing units (Houser & Player, 2007).

A&M's administration knew that the Rockefeller Foundation supported Carnegie. They helped her hire faculty and start a public health program. She wanted Florida A&M to have its own hospital and the school was awarded $50,000 for construction. A fundraising campaign provided the rest of the funding and a new, modern hospital was built in a few years. In her seven years at A&M, the program received national accreditation from the predecessor of today's National League for Nursing (NLN). This was a significant achievement because A&M was the first school in the state to receive this accreditation. It also was the only African American school in Florida run by an African American Dean that granted BSN degrees. The white schools only had Diploma programs and BSN programs were not established at the University of Florida and Florida State University until the early 1950s (Houser & Player, 2007).

Carnegie continued to experience racial discrimination and segregation. She was praised for her clinical rotation plan at a meeting of the Florida State Board of Nurse Examiners. The meeting was held at a hotel and she had to eat alone at a far table for lunch. She was humiliated, but stayed to prevent sanctions against her program and students. No one protested and she couldn't bring herself to participate in the afternoon discussions. When the University of Florida hosted its 25th anniversary celebration in 1981, Carnegie stated "I was invited as a guest and was cited for having pioneered baccalaureate nursing education in the state of Florida.... Times and people do change" (Houser & Player, 2007, p. 52).

Carnegie also pioneered the inclusion of African American graduate nurses in nursing professional organizations. Prior to the early 1940s, African American nurses in Florida couldn't join the Florida State Nurses Association or ANA. After 1942, African American nurses were allowed to join the Florida State Nurses Association and pay dues, but not have a voice or active participation in the organization. In 1946, the President of the Florida Association of Colored Graduate Nurses (FACGN) was invited to attend one session of the Florida State Nurses Association (FSNA) and the FSNA President was invited to attend one session of FACGN. Slight progress was being made. In 1947, both groups met in Daytona on opposite ends of town. For the first time, all African American nurses were invited to attend the joint program of FSNA and the Florida State League of Nursing Education. African American nurses had a voice in the educational issues presented. Carnegie had been elected President of FACGN and she became the voice of African American nurses throughout the state (Houser & Player, 2007).

In 1948, Elizabeth Carnegie presented the keynote address at the Florida Nurses Association's Convention. She would present the keynote address again to the same group 50 years later. In 1949, Carnegie was elected to the Board of Directors of FSNA for a one-year term. She was reelected the next year for three more years. Since African American nurses could join the state nurses' association, the FACGN dissolved in 1950. At first, there was a physical separation between African American and white nurses when they attended FSNA meetings. That didn't last long and soon seating was fully integrated (Houser & Player, 2007).

Another important milestone for Elizabeth Carnegie came in 1949. As FACGN President, she was invited to attend the International Council of Nurses meeting in Stockholm. Her members paid to send her and defrayed her expenses for the trip. While there, she participated in a study tour of six countries and reported on the ICN meeting at the FSNA Convention (Schorr & Zimmerman, 1988).

A new chapter in Carnegie's life began in 1953 when she moved to New York as an assistant editor for the *American Journal of Nursing*. She was now an African American nursing leader nationally. Racial discrimination followed her to New York when she tried to rent an apartment by her office and was told that the renting agent didn't rent to African Americans. Finally, she bought a home in Queens with financial help from a relative. For the rest of her career, Elizabeth Carnegie would be a leader in nursing journalism and writing for publication. Her rise in her new endeavors was meteoric. In three years, she was promoted to Associate Editor of *Nursing Outlook* with responsibility for the educational content of the publication. Carnegie was the first African American nurse to hold an editorial position and by 1970, she was Senior Editor of *Nursing Outlook* (Houser & Player, 2007).

Carnegie's influence in the nursing profession spread and she traveled nationally and internationally to influence change for minorities. She still wanted a doctorate and enrolled in the Graduate School of Public Administration at NYU to pursue this goal. In 1973, she attained her PhD, and her dissertation—*Disadvantaged Students in RN Programs*—was published by NLN. After her graduation, she became the Editor of Nursing Research, a position she held until her retirement (Carnegie, 1991).

Elizabeth Carnegie spent 25 years in nursing publications, and her editorials encouraged advanced education for nursing minorities. She also was active in organizations to promote funding for scholarships for minority nurses. As a member of the Board of Directors for Nurses Educational Funds, she earmarked funds for the Mary Elizabeth Carnegie Scholarship to support an African American doctoral student. When ANA received a grant to fund minority nurses seeking PhDs, she was appointed to the Minority Program Advisory Committee. Subsequently, she became chair of this group and it funded more than 200 nurses in doctoral preparation (Carnegie, 1991).

Carnegie also fostered participation by African American nurses in clinical research. After her induction, she started an endowment fund at the American Nurses Foundation to support the involvement of African American nurses in research. Howard University also recognized her with an annual M. Elizabeth Carnegie Research Conference that is international in scope (Houser & Player, 2007).

She continued her interest in education, publication, and research after retirement from *Nursing Research* by starting her own consulting firm. In this role, Carnegie traveled widely to consult with schools, present guest lectures, and conduct workshops about writing research for publication. Her popularity continued to grow as she made what she considered her greatest contribution to nursing: a book about the history of African Americans in nursing titled *The Path We Tread: Blacks in Nursing*. Initially, she had difficulty getting the book published, but it was a great success, resulting in television and radio appearances, speaking engagements, and book signings across the United States. Mary Elizabeth Carnegie earned numerous accolades and awards during her career, but she considered this book her crowning achievement (Schorr & Zimmerman, 1988). Carnegie used her writing to advocate changes in nursing education and practice, as Florence Nightingale did in her *Notes on Nursing* (Cook, 1913a).

She was recognized in a legislative resolution by the New York State Senate on May 22, 1986: "Resolved that this legislative body pause in its deliberations to honor Mary Elizabeth Carnegie for her contributions to the field of nursing as a nurse practitioner, educator, and author, and be it further resolved that this legislative body congratulate Mary Elizabeth Carnegie on her new book, *The Path We Tread: Blacks in Nursing*" (Houser & Player, 2007, p. 59).

Mary Elizabeth Carnegie had overcome racial discrimination and segregation through her lifetime contributions to nurses and the nursing profession. The legislative resolution was a fitting tribute to this crusader for national equality for African American nurses.

Implications for Nurse Leaders Today and in the Future
Contribution to Professional Literature

Elizabeth Carnegie was an expert on writing for publication and she realized the important role that professional literature could play in nursing progress and her campaign for equality of African American nurses (Schorr & Zimmerman, 1988). Florence Nightingale's approach to writing was "as a means to action" (Cook, 1913a, p. 474) and was typified by her book that established the basis for modern nursing: *Notes on Nursing* (Cook, 1913a).

Nurse leaders write reports, evaluations, schedules, memos, and requests for staffing, supplies, and equipment on a daily basis. However, they often don't consider their capability in writing for publication and that also must be considered as an aspect of their role. Nurse leaders can add to the profession's body of knowledge by sharing their own knowledge and expertise. Although research articles are always welcome, a well-written perspective about a clinical topic will be valuable to readers who are seeking information that they can use in their practice.

Many nurse leaders are unsure how to write an article for publication even if they have important clinical or leadership material to disseminate. Begin by selecting an appropriate journal for the article. Read the magazine's submission requirements and follow them carefully. Focus on clearly describing the topic and explaining its relevance and benefit to the profession. Once the idea for the article has been accepted for publication, it is time to begin writing the manuscript.

Here are techniques for improving the manuscript's quality based on Susan Gennaro's editorial in the July 2014 *Journal of Nursing Scholarship*:

1. Read paragraphs aloud to be certain sentences are not too long and rewrite sentences if needed for clarity. "Brevity improves clarity" (Gennaro, 2014, p. 217).
2. Let family and friends read the manuscript. Revise it if they cannot clearly understand the manuscript.
3. Ask colleagues to read and analyze the manuscript. Have them focus on quality and honestly identify any flaws.
4. Make time to write a priority and know ethical guidelines related to publication.
5. Develop a timeline for the manuscript and ensure that time dedicated to writing is not interrupted.
6. Use experts for literature searches and data analysis.

Nurse leaders today can learn from Carnegie and Nightingale's example. They must share their ideas in writing with professional colleagues to change and improve the nursing profession as their two predecessors did. They will be proud of the results.

— 14 —

Susie Walking Bear Yellowtail

Grandmother of American Indian Nurses

(January 27, 1903–December 1981)

Susie's Story

Susie Walking Bear was a member of the Apsáalooke (Crow) nation and was born on a reservation near Pryor, Montana, to an Apsáalooke father and a Sioux mother. As a child, she was orphaned at age 12 and attended a boarding school on the Apsáalooke reservation there (Montana Historical Society [MHS], n.d.). Students at mission boarding schools were required to adopt the English language and customs and forget their native languages, values, and culture. In Walking Bear's case, this didn't happen. She maintained her Apsáalooke character and customs and succeeded in the mission school by translating for other students as the only pupil who spoke English. Soon, her missionary foster parents moved with her to Oklahoma. After briefly attending a Baptist school there, she was sent by her guardian, Mrs. C. A. Field, to Northfield Seminary in Massachusetts. While Mrs. Field paid her tuition, Susie worked as a maid and babysitter to pay for her lodging and food (Ferguson, 2014).

After graduation, Walking Bear enrolled at Boston City Hospital's School of Nursing and graduated with honors in 1923. After finishing her training at Franklin County Public Hospital in Greenfield, Massachusetts, Walking

Bear became the first Apsáalooke registered nurse in the United States (Ferguson, 2014).

Walking Bear returned to the reservations to dedicate her life to serving Native Americans, first as a private duty and school nurse in Oklahoma, then as a home care nurse in Minnesota for the Chippewas there. In addition to conventional nursing practices, Walking Bear used Native American remedies to care for her patients (Voda, 2012). Walking Bear returned to the Apsáalooke Reservation in Montana and married Tom Yellowtail, a fellow Apsáalooke and religious leader, in 1929. Tom provided spiritual support for her throughout their life together, and family life was always her first priority. Their family grew to encompass a son, two daughters, two adopted sons, numerous tribally adopted sons, dozens of grandchildren, and great-grandchildren. Susie Yellowtail was deeply religious with a hearty laugh and a lively sense of humor (MHS, n.d.). These characteristics would be invaluable in both her personal life and her nursing career.

From 1929 to 1931, Yellowtail worked at the Bureau of Indian Affairs Hospital on the reservation. The experience outraged her. She observed blatant discrimination against Native American patients that included forcible sterilization of Apsáalooke women without their consent (Childs, 2012). She was not able to sit idly by while such atrocities occurred. She began a lifetime battle for change in her role as a healthcare advocate for Native Americans (American Society of Registered Nurses, 2007).

Florence Nightingale wrote in 1859 that

> *the most important practical lesson that can be given to nurses is to teach them what to observe-how to observe-what symptoms indicate improvement-what the reverse-which are of importance-which are of none-which are the evidence of neglect-and of what kind of neglect. (Nightingale, 1992, p. 59)*

Susie Yellowtail embraced this philosophy. From 1930 to 1960, She traveled to reservations throughout the United States to assess injustices to Native Peoples as a representative of the U.S. Public Health Service (MHS, n.d.). One of her assessments revealed that gravely ill Navajo children died on their mothers' backs during a walk of 20 miles or more to reach one of five hospitals serving 160,000 Navajo. She also provided midwifery services to Native American and non–Native American women in the Little Horn

Valley for 30 years (ANA, 2015c). Yellowtail realized that she had to become active in healthcare policy groups to advocate for healthcare equality for Native American tribes. She joined health advisory boards on a state level and soon was recognized by national health policy leaders for her work (Jennings, 2012).

Yellowtail was appointed to the Montana Advisory Committee on Vocational Education and her sense of humor and honesty opened doors for her as well as earned the respect of political leaders. She and Tom were part of a group sent by the State Department to Europe and the Middle East as goodwill ambassadors in the 1950s to promote understanding of Native American cultures (American Society of Registered Nurses, 2007).

Susie Yellowtail continued to advocate for reforms in the Indian Health Service. She documented her findings from her travels on reservations—children dying without access to medical care, women sterilized without their consent, and tribal elders unable to convey their health concerns to doctors. She recommended that traditional tribal elders participate in the care of Native American patients and encouraged creation of the Community Health Representatives Outreach Program on reservations (Ferguson, 2014). She became the spokeswoman for Native Americans on the reservations, advocating for expanded access to care, better health care, and improved living conditions (Ferguson, 2014). In 1962, she was recognized with the President's Award for Outstanding Nursing Health Care (Jennings, 2012).

Yellowtail's focus was making Native Americans strong and healthy and influential people listened to her because she spoke with confidence based on extensive knowledge. Native Americans trusted her because she promoted their culture and demonstrated her pride and devotion to their community. She served for years on the Apsáalooke Tribal Education and Health Committees as well as on boards of directors for many Native American-related associations and agencies (MHS, n.d.). In the 1970s, she influenced national Native American policy by her appointment to President Nixon's Council on Indian Health, Education and Welfare and the Federal Indian Health Advisory Committee. These appointments enabled Yellowtail to advocate nationally for the health needs of Native Americans (American Society of Registered Nurses, 2007; Jennings, 2012).

Susie Yellowtail also encouraged Native Americans to become nurses and founded the American Indian Nurses Association, which was the first professional association for Native American nurses. Her influence resulted in tribal and government funding for Native Americans entering the nursing profession. In 1978, she received a unique accolade when she was named "Grandmother of American Indian Nurses" by the American Indian Nurses Association (American Society of Registered Nurses, 2007). She always dressed as an Apsáalooke and practiced their religion to show pride in her heritage and serve as a conduit between Native Americans and non–Native Americans. Susie Yellowtail was a unique public servant whose wit, wisdom, and fortitude resulted in improved conditions for Native Americans (MHS, n.d.).

In 2002, Susie Yellowtail was inducted into the American Nurses Association Hall of Fame (ANA, 2015c). She is also enshrined in the Gallery of Outstanding Montanans in the Capitol Rotunda in Helena, Montana (Ferguson, 2014). Susie was a remarkable nurse and Apsáalooke woman who didn't seek honors. She was the voice for people who didn't have their own and exemplified commitment to children's well-being. She wanted to create a children's home and orphanage on the reservation, but died before realizing this goal (Ferguson, 2014). Yellowtail devoted her life to improving the treatment of Native Americans, including improved social services, educational opportunities, and health care that respected Native American rights. Her accomplishments were numerous, but more remains to be done. Funding is limited for Native American health care, social services, and education, and infant mortality remains high. Other nurses who will speak for the tribes must continue Yellowtail's legacy as advocates for improved health care and living conditions on the reservations (Voda, 2012).

The best tribute to Susie Walking Bear Yellowtail came from the Montana Historical Society: "Susie Walking Bear Yellowtail was an extraordinary Native American Leader. She nourished—physically, educationally and spiritually—all those around her" (MHS, n.d.). That is special recognition for a truly special person.

Implications for Nurse Leaders Today and in the Future
Importance of Assessment

Susie Yellowtail and Florence Nightingale both knew the importance of assessment (observation) and fought to improve people's lives and well-being (Voda, 2012; Nightingale, 1992). Today's nurse leaders also use assessment in their leadership activities to assess their units and service lines as well as other aspects of organizational performance. They base their assessments on Standard 1 of ANA's Standards of Practice: "The registered nurse collects pertinent data and information relative to the healthcare consumer's health or the situation" (ANA, 2015b, p. 53).

The first step in the assessment process involves data collection. Today, numerous tools are available to nurse leaders that enable them to take actions that support the organization's strategic plan. These tools include "clinical decision support systems (computerized data aggregation, assessment, interpretation...) and collective analytics (data integration, multisystems applications/correlation, and iterative/comprehensive implementation approaches) to inform appropriate action" (Porter-O'Grady, 2015, p. 25). These large data sources each have steps and actions illustrating their application to future organization actions by "big-data analytics" (Porter-O'Grady, 2015, p. 25). In step two of the assessment process, data calculations help nurse leaders "identify patterns and variances" (ANA, 2015b, p. 54) to address in their planning process, as stated in Standard 2 of Nursing Standards of Practice: "The registered nurse analyzes assessment data to determine actual or potential diagnoses, problems, and issues" (ANA, 2015b, p. 55).

Yellowtail and Nightingale used assessment data to improve the lives of Native Americans in the United States and English soldiers in the Crimea respectively (Childs, 2012; Cook, 1913a). Today's nurse leaders use assessment data to improve nursing practice at the unit and service line level. They also use assessment data to improve patient outcomes on the organizational level by following the other ANA Standards of Practice (ANA, 2015b, pp. 57–66):

> *Standard 3*—"The registered nurse identifies expected outcomes for a plan individualized to the healthcare consumer or the situation."
>
> *Standard 4*—"The registered nurse develops a plan that prescribes strategies and alternatives to attain expected, measurable outcomes."
>
> Standard 5—"The registered nurse implements the identified plan."
>
>> *Standard 5A*—"The registered nurse coordinates care delivery."
>>
>> *Standard 5B*—"The registered nurse employs strategies to promote health and a safe environment."
>
> *Standard 6*—"The registered nurse evaluates progress toward attainment of goals and outcomes."

Data assessment is particularly important in the diagnosis and evaluation phases for today's nurse leaders as it was for Susie Yellowtail in her quest to improve Native American lives by consulting with national leaders, recommending action plans, and evaluating results (Voda, 2012; Jennings, 2012). Nurse leaders have numerous data sources and their assessment skills use these resources to consult with other leaders and achieve results that enhance nursing practice in the unit and service line and patient outcomes in the organization.

~ *15* ~

Madeleine Leininger
Founder of Transcultural Nursing

(July 13, 1925–August 10, 2012)

Madeleine's Story

Madeleine Leininger was born in Nebraska in a family of five children with strong religious, family, and community values. As a child, she was influenced to become a nurse by her aunt, who was often hospitalized for congenital heart disease. Her aunt told Leininger "nursing is the most wonderful profession. You can help people when they need you most" (Schorr & Zimmerman, 1988, p. 188). After her aunt's death, Leininger's mother took in her sister's five sons to raise with her own five children. Leininger inherited her father's determination, commitment, and work ethic as well as her mother's sense of humor and enjoyment (Schorr & Zimmerman, 1988).

Since the family didn't have money for further education, Leininger and her sister entered the Cadet Nurse Corps in 1945 and the diploma program at St. Anthony's School of Nursing in Denver, Colorado (Schorr & Zimmerman, 1988; McFarland, 2006). Leininger thrived during her three years at St. Anthony's and was elected president of her nursing class. She effected positive changes and developed leadership skills in this position. Her experience showed her that anything valued or considered beneficial for people should be embraced. After graduation in 1948, Madeleine Leininger knew that she needed further education (Schorr & Zimmerman, 1988).

In 1950, she graduated from Mount St. Scholastica College (now Benedictine College) in Atchison, Kansas, with a BS in biological science and a minor in philosophy and humanistic studies (George, 2005; McFarland, 2006). Leininger worked as an instructor, staff nurse, and head nurse on the medical–surgical unit at St. Joseph's Hospital in Omaha and became Director of Nursing Service (DNS) there. She was interested in mental health nursing and opened a new psychiatric unit where she served as administrator, educator, therapist, and facilitator of multidisciplinary services (Schorr & Zimmerman, 1988). Education was Leininger's passion and she attended Creighton University in Omaha for advanced study in nursing administration, nursing curriculum development, and tests and measurements (McFarland, 2006).

In 1954, Leininger graduated with her MSN in psychiatric nursing from Catholic University in Washington, DC. At that time, the College of Health at the University of Cincinnati was seeking someone to begin the first graduate program in children's psychiatric nursing in the world. Leininger was up to the challenge and introduced the role of the clinical nurse specialist (CNS) in psychiatric nursing there. In addition to her responsibilities directing this graduate nursing program, she directed the Therapeutic Psychiatric Nursing Center at the university hospital (McFarland, 2006).

Leininger observed participant experiences in a Cincinnati child guidance center and saw that there were differences in how members of diverse cultures sought care. She believed these differences were cultural and resulted in disparities in treatment. The outcome was inadequate care for children from these cultures. Then, she met a person who would have a lasting impact on her life, career, and the nursing profession. Margaret Mead, the famous anthropologist, was a visiting professor at the University of Cincinnati and she challenged residents in child psychiatry to consider cultural implications in caring for these children. In her words: "On what basis are you making this diagnosis? What do you know about the cultural backgrounds of these children? How can you make an accurate diagnosis and attempt to help these children without cultural information?" (Schorr & Zimmerman, 1988, p. 189). Madeleine Leininger found her mentor and accepted Mead's challenge to study anthropology. It was an opportunity to study cultures in-depth and learn how to accurately interpret clients' behavior (Schorr & Zimmerman, 1988).

In 1959, Madeleine Leininger enrolled in the doctoral program in cultural, social, and psychological anthropology at the University of Washington. Cultural factors in diagnosis and treatment were unknown and other students didn't have the same interests. During her six years of study for her PhD, Leininger projected theories and methodologies that would make nursing a transcultural (influence of behavior by cultural values and beliefs) discipline. As she gained knowledge of religions, family relationships, political viewpoints, values, education, technology, and economics, Leininger learned how focused nursing was on Anglo-Saxon experiences. She found differences in caring, health, and well-being practices between Western and non-Western cultures. She began to develop her theory of culture care and the importance of using research and theory to help nurses and nursing students understand and practice in care, health, and illness (Schorr & Zimmerman, 1988; McFarland, 2006).

Leininger refined her theory during the next decade to develop a new field of study and practice that linked nursing and anthropology, called transcultural nursing. She identified common areas of knowledge and research interests between anthropology and nursing. She also encouraged nurses to pursue graduate education and practice in anthropology and by the mid-1960s had prepared nearly 5,000 nurses in classes, workshops, and degree programs in transcultural nursing. Leininger wanted her theory to describe, explain, interpret, and predict all cultures encountered in nursing. She established her own courses, programs, and field studies in transcultural nursing and introduced it in five major schools of nursing in the 1960s beginning with the University of Colorado in 1966 (Schorr & Zimmerman, 1988).

Madeleine Leininger was Professor of Nursing and Anthropology in 1966 at the University of Colorado when she developed her first transcultural nursing course. This was the first joint appointment in the United States of a nursing professor with another discipline. From there, she started and served as director of the first nurse scientist (PhD) program in 1969 at the University of Washington at Seattle where she established the Research Facilitation Office and guided the first nurses to PhDs in transcultural nursing. Then, Leininger became Dean and Professor of Nursing at the College of Nursing and Adjunct Professor of Anthropology at the University of Utah where she began the first master's and doctoral programs in transcultural nursing at the university. In 1981, Leininger became Professor of Nursing, Adjunct Professor of Anthropology, and Director of Transcultural Nursing Offerings at Wayne State University in Detroit. She stayed there until her semiretirement in 1995. During that time, she was Director of the Center for Health Research for five years where she mentored students in field research on transcultural nursing (McFarland, 2006).

She studied 14 different cultures as she developed her theory of cultural care diversity (difference in beliefs, values, and meanings between different cultures) and universality (common beliefs, values, and meanings). Her first field experience was with the Gadsup people of New Guinea. She lived with them two years, performing an ethnographic (study of individual cultures) and ethnonursing (beliefs, values, and practices about nursing care belonging to a specific culture) study of two of their villages. Leininger's passion ignited itself in others. She frequently was asked to consult on the cultural problems encountered by nurses to address conflict and stress about cultural rights. She discovered that there was greater resistance to transcultural nursing in areas with many different cultures and more openness in areas with few different cultures (Schorr & Zimmerman, 1988; McFarland, 2006).

Transcultural nursing became a global phenomenon and nurses overseas sought Leininger for advice. When Russian sailors were stranded in Tahiti, she helped the nurses there provide culture care for them. She also was one of the first nurse leaders to use qualitative research methods and taught these methods at universities worldwide. Her ethnonursing qualitative research methodology is the best method to discover the insider (emic) and outsider (etic) views of different cultures. It was the first nursing research method to examine cultural phenomena and complex care and is a holistic approach that is easy to use once learned. This methodology relates well to nursing and provides new insights about care, health, and well-being. Leininger's research was significant and resulted in transcultural nursing content and ideas to advance the discipline and profession of nursing (McFarland, 2006).

She contributed significantly to both nursing and anthropology and consulted for service and educational organizations after leaving academia. Leininger's interests were wide-ranging, including nursing theories, ethical nursing dilemmas, comparative education, administration, qualitative research methods, the future of nursing and health care, and nursing leadership. She founded the Transcultural Nursing Society and initiated the *Journal of Transcultural Nursing* as its first editor. She established the National Research Care Conference to study human caring phenomena. Leininger also established the committee on Nursing and Anthropology with the American Anthropological Association. Her literary contributions were impressive. She wrote or edited more than 27 books and published more than 200 articles and 45 book chapters as well as serving on editorial boards for several publications (McFarland, 2006).

Madeleine Leininger received numerous honors and awards as well as several honorary degrees. She was recognized by the American Academy of Nursing, the American Anthropology Society, and the Society for Applied Anthropology for her many contributions to both professions. Her assumption that care is the essence of nursing is now widely recognized and appreciated. (McFarland, 2006). Florence Nightingale and her example caring for soldiers in the Crimea would have supported Leininger's journey to establish care as the essence of nursing. Her caring extended to communication with the soldiers' loved ones at home, as evidenced by a letter she received from a soldier's sister: "It is great consolation to know that both his soul and body were so kindly cared for" (Cook, 1913a, p. 239).

Madeleine Leininger's identification of a major deficit in provision of nursing care related to culture care resulted in a defined pathway to address gaps caused by that deficit (McFarland, 2006; George, 2005). In her own words, "the combined nursing and anthropological perspective has provided me with special meanings and given me many challenges" (Schorr & Zimmerman, 1988, p. 192). These special meanings and challenges resulted in a new nursing theory that has been tested in clinical research and practice to result in culturally competent nursing care.

Implications for Nurse Leaders Today and in the Future
Caring and Culture

Caring is not a new concept, but Leininger's linkage of caring and culture established new relationships between nurses and clients. Her development of transcultural nursing carried Nightingale's emphasis on care to new heights and established a scientific discipline based on culture care (Cook, 1913a; McFarland, 2006). Today's nurse leaders should use these concepts to enhance their own and their staff members' cultural competence by looking at the patterns of structure of various cultures in their service areas (McFarland, 2006). Language translation services are helpful, but nurse leaders and other nurses must demonstrate awareness of the foundations of all cultures in the community. This includes incorporating in daily practice "12 community essentials (the foundation of all cultures) whenever possible" (Killen, 2013, p. 44).

These essentials include (Killen, 2013, p. 44):

1. "Locale: Where's the person from?"
2. "Communication: What's the most common language spoken in the home?"
3. "Family roles: Who's the one that makes healthcare decisions?"
4. "Work issues: Does economy play a role in healthcare?"
5. "Biocultural ecology: What types of ethnic issues may occur, such as race-specific diseases?"
6. "High-risk behaviors: Does this culture have practices detrimental to physical health?"
7. "Nutrition: What's the meaning of food to this culture, and what's the food choice at home?"
8. "Pregnancy and childbirth practices: What are the views on childbirth and pregnancy? Are there any customs that would make the patient uncomfortable if not performed?"
9. "Death rituals: What's the view of death, preparation for burial, and bereavement practices for family?"
10. "Spirituality: What are the behaviors that give meaning to life, including prayer and faith?"
11. "Healthcare practices: How does this culture view health, sickness, medicine, and healing?"
12. "Healthcare practitioners: What type of healthcare provider does this culture normally seek?"

There are many approaches to enhance nurses' practice when caring for members of a different culture. Presentations are helpful, but the information may not be readily accessed later when a patient from another culture arrives for care. It is important to remember that cultural care values the person's beliefs, values, and practices and continues throughout healing or preparation for death (McFarland, 2006). Killen described use of a cultural preference card system for patients to complete related to "the 12 community essentials" (Killen, 2013, p. 44) and for nurses to reference in providing culturally appropriate care. The nurse leader may choose to use this system or another one to support patients and nurses as they take this journey together. The nurse leader also role-models behavior in interactions with staff nurses and patients to reinforce Madeleine Leininger's assumption that the essence of nursing is care (McFarland, 2013).

— *16* —

Virginia Henderson
First Lady of Nursing

(November 30, 1897–March 19, 1996)

Virginia's Story

Virginia Henderson was the fifth of eight children and spent most of her childhood in Virginia because her father practiced law in Washington, DC. She attended her uncle's school for boys there along with her sister and aunt (WhyIWantToBeANurse.org, 2011). Her schooling was comprehensive, but no diploma was awarded. This delayed her acceptance to nursing school. Her interest in nursing grew from her desire to help wounded and sick military personnel in World War I and culminated in her enrollment in the Army School of Nursing in 1918 in Washington, DC, where she began to develop her definition of nursing. The students in the Army School of Nursing were treated like U.S. Military Academy cadets (Halloran, 2007). Henderson's basic nursing education was to learn by doing. Speedy performance, technical competence, and mastery of nursing procedures were valued. The approach to nursing care was impersonal and procedures, rather than ethics, were prized. She listened to lectures by physicians on disease, diagnosis, and treatment regimens. Nursing care was regimented and based on medical practice. That was dissatisfying to Henderson, who enjoyed her experiences with patients, but was concerned about a lack of role models for nursing students like herself. Students staffed hospitals, and clinical practice was a self-learned process. Her next education experience in psychiatric nursing was also disappointing. The focus was on disease and treatment with a lack of understanding about prevention and human relations skills (Lobo, 2005).

Courses were taught at Teachers College in Columbia University and Henderson found a mentor in Annie Goodrich (Halloran, 2007). Her pediatric experience at Boston Floating Hospital was more positive. The emphasis there was on family-centered care, continuity of care, and TLC (tender loving care). Although the facility was not task-oriented, there was little opportunity for parents to visit and lack of home assessment to determine child–family needs. Henderson's student experience at Henry Street exposed her to community nursing where patients' lifestyles were considered when providing care (Lobo, 2005). After graduation in 1921, she worked for two years at the Henry Street Settlement. She preferred this to hospital nursing and had an opportunity to explore her ideas about nursing, which was a rewarding experience (Lobo, 2005).

Henderson's first experience as an educator began in 1924 when she accepted the position of nurse educator at the Norfolk Protestant Hospital in Virginia. She was the first and only teacher in the school of nursing there (Halloran, 2007). After five years, she realized that she needed further knowledge to increase her effectiveness as an educator and enrolled at Teachers College to study humanities and sciences related to nursing. Her studies there helped her develop her analytical and inquiring approach to nursing (Lobo, 2005). Except for a brief period of employment at Strong Memorial Hospital in Rochester, Henderson completed her bachelor's and master's degrees at Teachers College with support from a Rockefeller Scholarship (Halloran, 2007).

Now, Virginia Henderson's career evolved as a nursing instructor at Teachers College for the next 16 years. Her focus was on clinical courses that emphasized the use of analytical process. Her reputation was growing and students were attracted to her courses (Lobo, 2005; WhyIWantToBeANurse. org, 2011). During her years at Columbia, she implemented several ideas in her medical–surgical courses that changed nursing practice. These included patient-centered care, nursing problem-solving methodology, field experience, family follow-up care, and chronic illness care. She utilized these approaches in establishing nursing clinics and encouraged multidisciplinary care coordination (Lobo, 2005).

In 1939, she was asked to update the fourth edition of Bertha Harmer's book *The Textbook of the Principles and Practice of Nursing*, which became a standard reference for many schools of nursing (WhyIWantToBeANurse. org, 2011). From 1948 to 1953, Henderson used her royalties from this edition for financial support while she completely revised this textbook to reflect her definition of nursing:

> *The unique function of the nurse is to assist the individual, sick or well, in the performance of those activities contributing to health or its recovery (or to peaceful death) that he would perform unaided if he had the necessary strength, will, or knowledge and to do this in such a way as to help him gain independence as rapidly as possible. (Tomey & Alligood, 2006, p. 55)*

Her textbook was used in hospital nursing schools in North America and standardized nursing practice (Halloran, 2007).

In 1953, Henderson's career in nursing research advanced when she joined the Yale School of Nursing as Research Associate to perform a critical review of nursing research. She found that most nursing research studied nurses rather than nursing care. Her editorials in professional journals stimulated more clinically focused nursing research. She saw a deficit of organized literature as a base for clinical studies and began a project to interpret nursing literature. This resulted in the *Nursing Studies Index*, a four-volume annotated index about nursing's historical, biographical, and analytical literature from 1900 to 1959. This project was acclaimed as Virginia Henderson's greatest contribution to nursing science (Tomey & Alligood, 2006; Halloran, 2007).

Her nursing need theory identified 14 basic human needs as the foundation for nursing care. She saw nursing as independent of medicine and identified three levels of nurse–patient relationships. These included the nurse as a substitute for the patient, the nurse as a helper to the patient, and the nurse as a partner with the patient. She advocated interdependence with physicians, other healthcare professionals, and the patient, with the patient contributing more as he or she gains independence. She focused on self-help concepts and her theory influenced the work of other nurse theorists. Henderson's major contributions to her profession included a definition of nursing, defining autonomous nursing functions, stressing interdependence to support the patient, and creating self-help concepts. Her theory represented a philosophy of nursing and she devoted her career to defining nursing practice and its unique functions (Tomey & Alligood, 2006; Lobo, 2005).

Virginia Henderson's nursing publications were widely translated and influential, making her the most acclaimed nursing writer since Florence Nightingale. Both women had something else in common: both hated to write and pushed themselves to accomplish the literary tasks they set for themselves (Halloran, 2007; Cook, 1913a). At 75, Henderson began the sixth edition of the *Principles and Practice of Nursing*. She and Gladys Nite led 17 collaborators in synthesizing the professional literature she had just indexed and the work took five years. This landmark publication was the first attempt at healthcare reform by nurses who advocated patient education and self-care to gain independence in health issues. She focused on individual and global levels and eliminated medical jargon so people could use it as a reference for their own or family's health needs. The book was an outstanding achievement (Halloran, 2007).

Virginia Henderson left Yale as Research Associate Emeritus at 75 and began a new career as a sought after speaker and international teacher. She shared her remarkable knowledge with a new generation (WhyIWantToBeANurse. org, 2011). She became a "nursing consultant to the world" (McBride, 1996, p. 23). Her awards and honorary degrees were numerous and she played a significant role in the nursing profession for more than 70 years as an educator, researcher, theorist, speaker, and author. She was also a genteel Southerner with a wry sense of humor and a knack for making others feel at ease. When nurses were nervous about being introduced to their icon, she cheerfully said, "I know that you have probably thought I've been dead for years" (McBride, 1996, p. 23). She was well dressed and gracious as well as interested in others. She engaged them in issues and discussions that stimulated her own inspired ideas. She exemplified caring and compassion throughout her life.

When Sigma Theta Tau's International Nursing Library (now the Virginia Henderson Global Nursing e-Repository) asked to use her name, Virginia Henderson

> *was only willing to permit use of her name if the electronic networking system to be developed would advance the work of staff nurses by getting to them current and jargon-free information wherever they*

were based. She was proud of that living testimonial to nursing excellence. (McBride, 1996, p. 23)

She truly was "the most famous nurse of the 20th century" (McBride, 1996, p. 23).

Implications for Nurse Leaders Today and in the Future
Patient-Centered Care

Virginia Henderson and Florence Nightingale both focused on nurse–patient relationships in their careers as reflected in their writings (Tomey & Alligood, 2006; Cook, 1913a). Today, the nurse–patient relationship is characterized by patient-centered care. Nurse leaders are familiar with the concept, but may be unsure of its impact in their care setting. RN engagement and retention are significant issues for healthcare leaders and a patient-centered care delivery model is a key component in nurses' satisfaction with their position as well as patient satisfaction. Both affect nurse leaders' units, service lines, and facilities financially. The cost of nurse turnover can be up to twice the nurse's salary and replacement cost can average $92,000 on a medical–surgical unit and up to $145,000 on a specialty unit (Hunter & Carlson, 2014). Hospital Consumer Assessment of Healthcare Providers and Systems (HCAHPS) scores are used to determine patients' view of the care they received and low HCAHPS scores result in decreased Medicare reimbursement through the Value-Based Purchasing Program (Hunter & Carlson, 2014).

The Joint Commission recognizes that "leaders must clearly articulate a hospital's commitment to meet the unique needs of its patients to establish an organizational culture that values effective communication, cultural competence, and patient- and family-centered care" (Hunter & Carlson, 2014, pp. 40–41). Patient-centered care has existed since Virginia Henderson created her nursing need theory (WhyIWantToBeANurse.org, 2011). Several principles describe patient-centered care (Hunter & Carlson, 2014, p. 41):

1. The patient and family must be at the center of "operational, quality, safety, and care structures."
2. Care delivery must focus "on the patient as a person."
3. Nurses and patients must interact closely and communicate with each other to adapt patient care to patient needs.
4. Nurses must become "guests in the patient's world".

5. Nurses must collaborate with patients and "partners in care" to ensure that patients and families are involved in every care decision so they can make informed decisions about their own care.

The nurse leader must facilitate these nursing practice changes by endorsing patient-centered care and ensuring that nurses receive support and education as they transition to their new roles. The nurse leader must use Henderson's third level of nurse–patient relationships—partnership with the patient—to reinforce its importance to nurses in delivering patient-centered care (Tomey & Alligood, 2006). This isn't just a financial necessity for health care. It's the right thing to do.

$$- \enspace 17 \enspace -$$

Luther Christman

Nursing Visionary

(February 26, 1915–June 7, 2011)

Luther's Story

Luther Christman's older brother died shortly after birth and two other siblings died in infancy. He was the first living child to parents who were polar opposites. His father was gentle and hard working. His mother was prejudiced, and her oldest son was a target for her abuse. She was Methodist and believed it was the only true faith. She despised Catholics and belonged to the local Ku Klux Klan, which burned crosses at Catholic homes in their small Pennsylvania community. Christman abandoned organized religion at 15 because of exposure to this prejudice. Elizabeth Christman physically abused her son from an early age, first with a leather razor strop and then with a cat-o'-nine-tails. His father was dominated by his wife and never protected Christman from her violence. His two younger sisters weren't physically battered and she loved his younger brother (Pittman, 2005).

Luckily, Christman's maternal grandmother was warm and affectionate toward him. She and her husband encouraged him to succeed in school and taught him the Golden Rule. His mother started him in school at age 4 because she wanted him to graduate at 16 and earn a living. At first, he couldn't keep up with the other students and was the smallest one in his class. As the years passed, he made friends and achieved scholastically. He participated in the school band, school plays, and the debate team. Christman also began writing poetry and developed an interest in art and biology. He worked throughout his teens selling newspapers and magazines and for a local baker. His mother took all the money he earned except for an occasional nickel or dime (Pittman, 2005).

The Methodist and Lutheran ministers suggested that Christman become a clergyman, but he wasn't interested. Then, the Methodist minister suggested a nursing career. He was dating Dorothy Black and didn't want to leave her. She agreed to become a nurse and they applied to two schools of nursing in Philadelphia—the Pennsylvania Hospital School of Nursing for Men and Methodist Hospital School of Nursing. Christman wasn't concerned about being a man in a women's profession. He knew this was an opportunity to earn a living while he learned and a chance to leave a negative home. In his words, "My mother was always putting me down and never wanted me to be successful but in spite of that [or because of it] I developed a passionate commitment to succeed" (Pittman, 2005, p. 37). Luther Christman survived his childhood and years later learned that his father loved him: "After my mother died my father opened up to me and I realized he adored me" (Pittman, 2005, p. 26).

Christman now embarked on a new chapter in his life as a trainee nurse at Pennsylvania Hospital School of Nursing for Men. New challenges awaited him there. After presenting a recommendation from his high school principal, he was interviewed and completed two days of clinical psychology tests and assessments. When he passed, he was accepted as a patient attendant for eight months until the start of classes. It was a probationary period that reduced 75 applicants to 30 who became student nurses. Christman, at 21, was the youngest in his class again. Only 8 men successfully completed the entire program and he was among them (Pittman, 2005).

Women nurses viewed men in nursing with suspicion and faculty was segregated. Christman confronted prejudice frequently during his training. Once he was in surgery and was told to leave the room because the woman patient had to be catheterized and a man who wasn't the doctor couldn't be present. When he protested, he was told he didn't understand the role of men in the profession. Christman had to pass obstetrics in his RN licensing exam, but men weren't welcome in OB nursing rotations.

Although firemen, policemen, and taxi drivers were trained for emergency deliveries, a male nursing student could not receive that training. Christman was refused this opportunity and told that "if [he] was ever seen anywhere near the delivery room, [he] would be dismissed immediately" (Pittman, 2005, p. 44). His only option was to study for the exam using textbooks. When he took the test, he was the first to complete it and he scored 98% with no clinical experience! The director of nursing who refused his request for training later became his supporter and gave him a recommendation (Pittman, 2015).

Before he graduated, a night supervisor position was available in a smaller hospital that interested Christman. When he interviewed, he asked when a day position would be available and was told the following: "Never, we would not allow our patients to know that we had a male nurse on staff" (Schorr & Zimmerman, 1988). He didn't take the position. He and Dorothy graduated in 1939 and married that December. He became a private duty nurse at Pennsylvania Hospital (Christman, 2015).

World War II changed Christman's life again. In December 1941, he was 24 and had a wife and infant son. His patriotic inclination was to serve in the Army Nurse Corps. There was one problem. The 1901 law establishing the Corps designated members as women. Never one to back down from a challenge, Christman wrote the surgeon general asking to serve at the front as a nurse. Men could only serve as noncommissioned orderlies, not as nurses. He was overqualified as a nurse and not allowed to attend Corps School so he was prohibited from that role. The Army was desperate for nurses, but men were assigned to non-nursing tasks and women were only allowed in base hospitals, not the front lines. Christman's letter to the surgeon general requesting posting as a nurse in the war zone received a terse response. He began a campaign to get men in the Nurse Corps by sending copies of his letter and the response to all U.S. Senators and 75% of the House of Representatives. His appeal became public and gained support from Congressional leaders (Pittman, 2005).

In the meantime, Christman was concerned about being drafted to a non-nursing post so he joined the U.S. Maritime Service as a "Pharmacist's Mate First Class" (Pittman, 2005, p. 16). Many nurses were opposed to men in the Corps because they feared that men would take over the officer positions created in 1942. The Pinnella County District Nurses Association publicly supported Christman and ANA sent a letter to the surgeon general without his knowledge requesting that male nurses have equal opportunities to serve. The surgeon general didn't want male nurses or African American female nurses commissioned and testified before several Congressional committees explaining his position. Then, the surgeon general introduced a bill to draft women nurses. The bill was subsequently dropped and efforts to commission male nurses stalled. Christman's campaign failed to achieve its objective and none of the 1,200 male nurses drafted were allowed to function as nurses. Men weren't accepted in the Nurse Corps until the Korean War. A bill by Senator Bolton eliminated discrimination against men as nursing officers and by 2005, over 30% of registered nurses in the Military Nurse Corps were men (Pittman, 2005; Schorr & Zimmerman, 1988).

After serving through the war at St. Petersburg, Florida, Christman and his family returned to Philadelphia where he wanted to pursue his BA in nursing. Two schools refused to admit him because he was a man. Then, he went to Temple University and was admitted with no problems. After graduation in 1948, he became a faculty member at the Cooper Hospital School of Nursing for the next five years (Christman, 2015). He honed his leadership and innovation skills there by focusing on organizational effectiveness and nurse productivity. He introduced ward clerks, automatic medication replacement, enlarged supply station, and messengers to remove nonclinical duties from the nurses. He also managed to upset the head nurses who didn't want to only care for patients. Christman learned valuable lessons about the importance of staff involvement in decision-making and how nurses resist change. When he was offered the position of associate administrator, he refused so he could stay in nursing (Schorr & Zimmerman, 1988).

By 1952, Luther Christman earned an MA in clinical psychology from Temple and moved to South Dakota in 1953 as Director of Nursing at Yankton State Hospital. The facility needed reform, but the attendants were embedded and resistant to change. He surveyed them to discover their three favorite and three least favorite assignments. Then, he assigned them to their least preferred duties. Three immediately resigned and the nurses, physicians, and professional staff initiated reforms using the practitioner-teacher model. The changes gained wide support, and Christman was appointed to the South Dakota Board of Nursing. He advocated nurse-physician teams to manage patients and believed nurses had the same accountability as physicians and had responsibility for quality of nursing care. He endorsed a primary nursing model that used aides as assistants to nurses rather than caregivers. He also promoted master's preparation for nurses and was appointed to the first national committee to examine this concept and make recommendations, a document later published by NLN (Schorr & Zimmerman, 1988).

Christman's next nursing position was as a nursing consultant for the Michigan Department of Mental Health from 1956 to 1963 (Christman, 2011). In his work to change the mental health system there, he promoted a unified model in psychiatric nursing. He also discovered that some nurses lobbied to have psychiatric aides licensed and educated like LPNs. He wanted scholarships for professional nurses instead and asked legislators to pass the aide bill, but not fund it. When that occurred, funding for nursing scholarships succeeded. During those years, Christman was active in ANA and NLN and enrolled in the doctoral program at Michigan State University. He also was elected president of the Michigan Nurses Association and coerced the Michigan Hospital Association to increase nurses' salaries. His success was measured by an increase in the number of nurses with active licenses from 14,000 to 21,000 (Schorr & Zimmerman, 1988).

Christman's next nursing position was as Associate Professor of Psychiatric Nursing at the University of Michigan at Ann Arbor in 1963 (Christman, 2011). Besides his appointment in the School of Nursing, he also held appointments in the Institute for Social Research and the Bureau of Hospital Administration. He collaborated with a colleague (Basil Georgopoulos) on a controlled field experiment to study the role of the nurse specialist and suggested changes to administration of hospitals. He also wrote Christman's Laws of Behavior:

> *We all want the world to be in our image. People cannot use knowledge they do not have. In every instance, given the choice between rationality and irrationality, people opt for irrationality and are rational only when forced to be. Most people under most circumstances will generally do what is right if they know what is right and if the temptation to err is not too great. (Schorr & Zimmerman, 1988, pp. 49–50)*

He completed his PhD in sociology and anthropology from Michigan State in 1965 with a dissertation on "perceptions resulting from vertical division of labor and its effect on organizational cohesion" (Sullivan, 2002, p. 12).

He was a visionary who proposed changes in the nursing profession that others did not contemplate. In 1964, Christman proposed the creation of the American Academy of Nursing. He also advocated for establishment of a BSN entry level and nurse practitioner programs in the face of opposition by nursing colleagues. The prejudice Luther Christman encountered earlier in his career reappeared at different times along with opportunities for success. His wry humor helped him deal with criticism because of his gender and his disappointment that nursing didn't adhere to affirmative action (Sullivan, 2002; Schorr & Zimmerman, 1988).

Christman's career was thriving. He became the Dean of Nursing at Vanderbilt University and Director of Nursing at Vanderbilt Hospital in 1967. It was the first time that a man was a nursing dean. Vanderbilt was an opportunity to develop a nurse practitioner program, but the nursing association opposed nurse practitioners, fearing these nurses would function as doctors. He gained the support of the Tennessee Medical Association, but nursing opposition resulted in the establishment of physician assistant programs (Sullivan, 2002). Christman's accomplishments at Vanderbilt offset this setback. He refined the practitioner–teacher model and obtained grant funding to develop nursing practice as an applied science and to improve education in behavioral sciences. Funding also improved the effectiveness of learning laboratories. As a result, student numbers increased and his proposal to integrate the education of graduate students—medical and nursing—created the foundation for advanced practice nursing. His concern for minorities in nursing resulted in him hiring the first African American women as faculty members at Vanderbilt (Palmer, 2011).

In spite of his triumphs at Vanderbilt, a meeting of deans of the Southern Regional Education Board demonstrated that prejudice against men in nursing still existed. After the meeting, a woman dean approached Christman and demanded to know how he—a man—had accomplished so much and told him that he should never have been allowed to outstrip women in nursing. He deflected her observations about his competence with humor, but the incident showed how much further male nurses had to go for acceptance in their own profession (Schorr & Zimmerman, 1988; Sullivan, 2002).

In 1968, a momentous occasion occurred in Christman's life and career. It happened when he was nominated for president of the American Nurses

Association. He met all the qualifications and had a wave of support, except for the board. Suddenly, a rumor swirled about his sexual orientation. For a husband and father of three, it seemed ridiculous. However, the rumor eroded his support and his candidacy failed (Pittman, 2005). Some of the nurses there believed that "no man should ever be elected president of the ANA" (Schorr & Zimmerman, 1988, p. 51). It represented a lost opportunity for him to attain a position to influence the progress of nursing (Sullivan, 2002).

In 1972, another momentous occasion was more positive for Christman and his vision of nursing. Rush University in Chicago hired him to help launch the school and develop dynamic nursing programs there. He opened the College of Nursing and Allied Health Services within one year at both undergraduate and graduate levels. He also served as VP of Nursing at Rush-Presbyterian-St. Luke's Medical Center, a joint appointment of service and nursing education. Christman was VP for Operations for both organizations. Rush gave him a chance to implement his vision for nursing. Since he believed nursing faculty members should be proficient practitioners, they spent two-thirds of their time in practice and were reimbursed at the same level for practice as medical faculty. Their salaries were paid from the nursing college budget to ensure excellent clinical education for Rush students (Sullivan, 2002).

The Rush Model, a unified approach to nursing education, research, and practice, included unit decentralization, a quality assurance program, primary nursing, levels of practice, the practitioner–teacher role, and self-governance by professional staff (Christman, 2011). Christman also implemented nurse practitioner and clinical doctoral programs at Rush as well as a combined DNSc/PhD degree program. At the time, NLN promoted education degrees for faculty and few clinical degrees were available (Sullivan, 2002).

While establishing these innovations in nursing, Luther Christman continued to encourage and support men in nursing. He helped establish the National Male Nurse Association in 1974 and revitalized it in 1980. The following year, it became the American Assembly for Men in Nursing (Christman, 2011). Throughout his career, he supported affirmative action strategies for men in nursing and actively encouraged schools to recruit men. Some schools adopted his approach while others refused to admit any men. Christman wasn't surprised. It was just another challenge to overcome (Sullivan, 2002).

He retired from Rush in 1987, but he didn't retire as an advocate for the profession he loved. He continued to address his view of nursing's problems, including solving the nursing shortage by actively recruiting men, addressing the need for highly skilled and educated professionals to provide care as technology advances, and making the baccalaureate degree the entry level to nursing practice while maintaining community colleges by offering lower division education courses there (Sullivan, 2002).

Luther Christman received numerous honorary degrees, awards and recognition. He was the first man admitted to the American Nurses Hall of Fame and designated a Living Legend by the American Academy of Nursing (Palmer, 2011). His vision for nursing has been validated and his ideas, once considered radical, are now accepted in nursing education and practice. His son was the only one of his three children to follow him into nursing, but he couldn't deal with discrimination and left the profession. Christman told an interviewer who asked why he stayed in nursing, "I wanted to change things. I was determined to change things and do them correctly" (Sullivan, 2002, p. 14). He had one trait in common with Florence Nightingale: both were reformers in nursing and health care (Cook, 1913a; Pittman, 2005).

Luther Christman is gone, but his legacy continues and his greatest contribution to nursing will be the day when the term 'male nurse' is replaced simply with 'nurse'.

Implications for Nurse Leaders Today and in the Future
Innovation

Luther Christman and Florence Nightingale both were visionaries who experimented with innovative changes in nursing—she in transformation of care in Liverpool workhouses; he in implementation of the Rush Model for Nursing in Chicago (Cook, 1913b; Christman, 2011). Today's nurse leaders cannot focus on the status quo. Nursing and health care are changing constantly and it is imperative that nurse leaders use innovative approaches in their roles to advance nursing in their facilities and as a profession. They need to begin by looking at productivity in a new way. Historically, healthcare organizations have defined productivity as "time spent in direct care at the bedside" (Altman & Rosa, 2015, p. 46). Time away from the bedside is classified as nonproductive. This narrow view doesn't promote innovation. Innovation is not a scheduled activity. It evolves from an opportunity to explore improved patient outcomes and increased quality of care that may occur as nurses assess, plan, and evaluate care or as they participate in education and committees (Altman & Rosa, 2015).

Nonproductive time or indirect care isn't a negative concept when used to seek improved patient and clinical outcomes. Today's nurse leaders have an unprecedented opportunity to guide nurses to influence "the primary mission of patient care and advancing nursing practice" (Altman & Rosa, 2015, p. 48). Nurses are capable of being innovators and change agents by creating unit changes that can result in improvements in patient care and organizational efficiency and effectiveness. Nurse leaders must encourage out-of-the-box thinking and provide nurses with the resources they need to encourage innovative solutions to nursing and healthcare problems.

A successful example of nursing innovation is based on collaboration of the Robert Wood Johnson Foundation and the Northwest Health Foundation to develop leadership and innovation skills of clinical nurses. Their Partners Investing in Nursing's Future grant enabled the American Association of Critical-Care Nurses (AACN) Clinical Scene Investigator (CSI) Academy to inspire clinical nurses in transforming nursing and health care. The 16-month program enlists a team of four clinical nurses who are guided by faculty, their CNO, and a mentor (leader) within their facility to investigate patient care issues, develop and implement a change project related to their clinical unit(s), and evaluate results of their actions. The program focuses on leadership, project management, and entrepreneurial skills. Education on healthcare policy is studied to learn its impact on nursing and how nursing influences the facility's financial outcomes. Participants also learn to use quality improvement data and perform financial analysis to determine how their change projects affect the organization's revenue stream. Since change doesn't occur in a vacuum, team members must enlist the support of peers for successful change. The clinical nurses' enhanced leadership skills involve how to engage stakeholders in the change process. This is vital in expanding project improvements to additional clinical areas. Although these nurses are still participating in patient care during the 16 months, they attend workshops, develop tools, review data, develop and implement their change project, and evaluate the financial impact of their project on the unit and organization. Their use of nonproductive time demonstrates that it can be as (or more) effective as direct care delivery (Altman & Rosa, 2015).

What innovations have occurred as a result of participation in the AACN CSI Academy and what are the financial results? These nurse-driven projects have been wide ranging, maintained, and adopted by other clinical units. Their outcomes have netted "more than $28 million of estimated savings for participating hospitals" (Altman & Rosa, 2015, p. 50). Their scope has included focus on early ambulation, delirium prevention, and nurse-sensitive indicators such as hospital-acquired pressure ulcers (HAPU), catheter-associated urinary tract infections (CAUTI), central line-associated bloodstream infections (CLABSI), and ventilator-associated pneumonia (VAP). Would this innovation have occurred during productive time providing patient care? That's a question impossible to answer at present, but there certainly is a case for using nonproductive time wisely that leaders must encourage for innovation to occur.

Nightingale's own words should guide nurse leaders to seek and promote innovation: "Never lose an opportunity of urging, a practical beginning, however small, for it is wonderful how often in such matters the mustard-seed germinates and roots itself" (Altman & Rosa, 2015, p. 50). Our healthcare system and nursing continue to evolve and nurse leaders must support nurses' efforts for innovation as well as developing their own as leaders of change. Remember that many of the 'radical' innovations advocated by Luther Christman are accepted nursing practices today and today's nurses and nurse leaders have opportunities to revolutionize their profession and health care itself for the future (Sullivan, 2002; Altman & Rosa, 2015).

— 18 —

Richard Carmona
Always a Nurse

(November 22, 1949–)

Rich's Story

Richard Carmona has had a stellar career that might never have happened. He was the first of four children of Puerto Rican parents to be born in the United States. Growing up in Harlem, he grew up in poverty in a family struggling to survive. His mother, Lucy, spoke French, German, Spanish, and English. She was a self-taught artist and musician who taught Carmona that he needed an education and that he could achieve anything. His father was frequently absent and worked sporadically. He was pleasant, but a poor communicator. As Carmona grew older, he became a substitute father for his two younger brothers and sister because they seldom saw his father. Both parents and his maternal grandmother drank and his mother and grandmother were chain smokers. Luckily, Rich Carmona had a protector—his paternal grandmother, or *Abuelita*, who taught her favorite grandchild Spanish and about his cultural heritage and personal responsibility. Maria Anglade Carmona emigrated from Puerto Rico by herself with 9 children and 18 stepchildren. The youngest was Carmona's father, Raoul (Mattson, 2005). Rich's abuelita was the neighborhood seamstress and community coordinator who cared for other immigrants by opening her home to them every Sunday. She was the stabilizing factor in her grandson's childhood and showed him the value of community service and helping others (Houser & Player, 2007).

When Carmona was six, his family became temporarily homeless and lived for 18 months with Abuelita in her tiny apartment. When they eventually found a roach-infested tenement apartment, Abuelita brought food and other necessities. The apartment was hot in the summer and cold in the winter and hot water was sporadic. Since the adults didn't have steady employment, hunger was a concern daily. As Carmona remembers, "it is hard to focus on homework or SAT exams when you are consumed with where the next meal will come from" (Houser & Player, 2007, p. 7). His mother smoked and drank in the evenings, but she also read to her children from library books and encyclopedias and quizzed them afterward. Carmona loved her and his grandmother, and their message was the same—that he should get an education and that he could be successful.

By sixth grade, their lessons fell on deaf ears. He developed skills to survive in his crime- and drug-infested neighborhood and those skills didn't include attending school and studying for good grades. He skipped classes and lacked interest in school. Abuelita died when he was 14 and his behavior remained unchanged. He enjoyed team sports and students were bussed to the Bronx to join teams. However, class attendance was necessary to join a team and he still was a truant. Carmona learned to sign in for homeroom and then he quietly left until it was time for practice. When his absences were discovered, he had to report to the counselor's office. The two counselors focused on helping him make better choices and persuaded the principal to give him chance after chance when his behavior recurred. His lack of academic progress caused Carmona to drop out in his senior year and he spent his days on the streets of Harlem with no thoughts for the future (Houser & Player, 2007).

There was one stabilizing influence in Carmona's life as a teenager. Her name was Diane Theresa Sanchez, the daughter of a NYPD detective whose family lived near Abuelita's apartment when he was 12. He enjoyed talking with Diane, whose family was primarily in law enforcement. At 15, Carmona coached her younger brother's football team and they began to talk again and developed a friendship that would blossom into love. Her mother liked Rich and fed him when her husband was at work. She also washed his clothes, separating white from dark colors to return them to their original shades. While Diane's mother was kind and caring, her father wanted nothing to do with Carmona, who he felt wasn't good enough for his daughter. He primarily ignored Rich until the night that Carmona took Diane to her senior prom. He borrowed money for the tux, corsage, and transportation and came to pick up Diane. Her father, Vinnie, brought out a box of his pistols and began cleaning them at the kitchen table while glaring at his unwelcome visitor. His meaning was clear especially when he ignored Carmona's greeting. Vinnie wouldn't accept him until 1971 when Diane and Rich married (Houser & Player, 2007).

Before their wedding, Carmona would be tested on another battlefield in Southeast Asia and finally see a purpose for his future. He was 17 and struggling to survive on the streets when he met another positive influence named Sal Hasson, a member of the Green Beret Special Forces. When Sal talked about his experiences at a local candy store, Carmona was fascinated. It was an opportunity to do something with his life, and he joined the Army in 1967. He passed the entrance exams and found himself at Fort Jackson, South Carolina, in boot camp. It was a revelation for a streetwise kid who had never followed rules. Boot camp was all about rules and discipline. He also had a firsthand view of racial discrimination that he hadn't seen in Harlem, including segregated drinking fountains, entrances, and transportation. It was the first time he experienced the effect of such prejudice and he never forgot it (Houser & Player, 2007).

Carmona wanted to join the Special Forces, but the path wasn't easy for a high school dropout. Over two years, he completed infantry training, parachute school, and earned his general equivalency diploma (GED). When he finally was accepted in the Special Forces, he was trained as a weapons and medical specialist, obtaining basic nursing skills that he would use within and after service. Carmona also learned life skills that he would use successfully later on. He acquired management, organizational, and strategic planning knowledge that enabled him to be proactive and willing to take risks (Houser & Player, 2007).

Carmona's newly acquired nursing skills were tested in the jungles of Vietnam in 1969. He delivered babies and became proficient at caring for "burns, traumatic injuries from explosions, gunshot wounds requiring surgery, infectious diseases, parasitic diseases, malnutrition, and sanitation for the village" (Houser & Player, 2007, p. 14). The experience trained Rich to recognize and treat public health problems caused by parasites and microorganisms.

In addition to his responsibilities as a medical specialist, Sgt. Richard Carmona also conducted Special Forces combat operations in his role as a weapons specialist. He demanded to participate in the rotation for combat missions within his 12-man team. His courage and leadership earned Rich numerous combat awards, including "the Bronze Star, two Purple Hearts, a Combat Medical Badge, the Vietnam Cross of Gallantry, and many other citations" (Houser & Player, 2007, p. 15). He gained lifelong friends and Diane faithfully communicated with him by daily letters, holiday care packages, and an annual birthday cake. She even met him in Hawaii for R&R (Houser & Player, 2007).

In 1970, Carmona returned to New York City and found another combat zone of violence, drugs, and casualties exacerbated by poverty and poor life choices. He knew the only way out for him was the education his mother and grandmother had advocated and he took advantage of the open enrollment program for Vietnam veterans with a GED from Bronx Community College (BCC) and became an A student (Mattson, 2005). He worked his way through school there as a part-time lifeguard, and one of his professors, Henry Hermo, remembers that Carmona "took others under his wing. When he came to BCC, he wasn't looking back, he was really looking forward. He was outstanding" (From High School Dropout to Surgeon General, 2002).

On September 4, 1971, Diane and Rich married and he finally received Vinnie's approval. In February 1974, the couple visited a friend of Carmona's from Vietnam in California and decided to move there. He transferred to finish his bachelor's degree at Long Beach's California State University. Then, he had to find a job. California permitted medics to take the RN licensing exam in the early 1970s based on the curriculum of the Special Forces. He passed the exam and found employment as an ED nurse while pursuing pre-med studies full-time. He wasn't fazed by the fact that he sometimes was the only male nurse in the hospital. He believed "the gender difference was a bi-directional learning experience that improved all players" (Houser & Player, 2007, p. 19).

Carmona was successful in ED as a nurse because many of the physicians there, who moonlighted in ED with little or no experience in trauma care, were former members of the military. They worked well with him because he was knowledgeable and could help triage patients. He used his skills as a medic and learned nursing skills from his fellow ED nurses. They educated him about "holistic care, collaboration, and interdisciplinary teamwork" (Houser & Player, 2007, p. 19). He also completed training on mobile intensive care nursing which combined ED and intensive care nursing skills to provide prehospital trauma care. He enjoyed nursing and drew on those skills as he became a physician and later as surgeon general (Mattson, 2005).

In 1976, Carmona began medical school at the University of California at San Francisco (UCSF). He met two other RNs there and they convinced the nursing and medical schools to collaborate and provide a nursing skills lab for medical students that gave them an opportunity to learn to write legible orders, how to take vital signs, how to chart, and most of all, basic nursing skills. The medical students gained a new perspective about the role and value of nurses (Houser & Player, 2007). He graduated in 1979 a year early at the top of his class. He won the University's Gold Cane Award as vale-dictorian (University of California, Department of Surgery, 2014). He also invited his parents to fly to San Francisco at his expense for the ceremony. He sent them tickets even though he didn't have much money. Neither came and he never succeeded in relocating them from their old neigh-borhood (Houser & Player, 2007). However, Carmona was determined to honor his parents and in 2000, the Carmona family established the Raoul & Lucy Carmona Memorial Scholarship, which was awarded to two first-year University of Arizona medical students. Rich's daughter, Carolyn Carmona Guillot, a critical care and trauma RN, presented the award (Mattson, 2005; Arizona Latin-American Medical Association, 2014).

Carmona's academic achievements mirrored his motivation to succeed. He completed his surgical residency at UCSF and an NIH fellowship in trauma, burns, and critical care (Mattson, 2005). In 1985, he was hired by the Tucson Medical Center to start its first trauma center and served as Director of Trauma Services there until his position was eliminated in 1993 when the program merged with the University Medical Center trauma program, much to his patients' dismay. He sued and won a public apology and confidential settlement. In 1995, he became CEO and Medical Director of Tucson's Kino Community Hospital and two years later was promoted to head of the Pima County Health System. He inherited a financially unstable public hospital that served an indigent population and ran huge deficits. Unable to stabilize the organization financially and without support from the county health commissioners, he resigned in July 1999 (Pederson & Garvey, 2002).

Carmona became a champion for bioterrorism preparedness when it wasn't a popular cause. After September 11, he became the leader in implementing bioterrorism and emergency-preparedness plans for southern Arizona. He also has been actively involved in public safety since he joined the Pima County Sheriff's Office in 1986 as a doctor, deputy sheriff, and SWAT team member. He sees both roles—doctor and lawman—as essential to protect public safety and continues to serve as department surgeon (Frank, 2002; Pima County Sheriff's Department, 2015).

Carmona's courage was tested under fire during the last decade of the 20th century. In 1992, a medevac helicopter crashed into the side of a mountain and he saved the survivor by hanging on a rope from another helicopter, pulling the paramedic to him, and carrying him to safety. In 1999, he drove past an accident scene while off duty and stopped to assist. An enraged driver was attacking a woman and shot at Carmona when he asked him to put down the gun. The man fired, grazing Carmona's forehead, and he fired back, killing him. The man had killed his father earlier in the day and Rich Carmona was recognized for saving bystanders' lives by the National Association of Police Organizations as a 'Top Cop' in 2002 (Pederson & Garvey, 2002; Pear, 2002; Frank, 2002). He also received the medical society 'Top Doctor' award the same year (Houser & Player, 2007).

His time as surgeon general was no less tumultuous. After his appointment in 2002, he found himself at odds with the administration. He released an updated report on the dangers of secondhand smoke and recommended that an environment without exposure to secondhand smoke become a national priority (Department of Health and Human Services, 2006). A report on global health did not fare as well. Carmona wanted to share the most important global health challenges with average Americans and explain why they should care. The head of the Office of Global Health Affairs wanted the report to focus on the accomplishments of the administration and didn't want global warming mentioned. The report was never published and Carmona left office in July 2006. He remained quiet for several months before speaking out about the politicizing of the position. He and his two predecessors testified before the House Oversight and Government Reform Committee and all three agreed that the surgeon general should advocate for scientific evidence, not political causes (Harris, 2007; Lee, 2007).

His nursing background was beneficial during his term as surgeon general and he contacted nursing organizations shortly after his appointment to involve nurses in disaster planning and response. He collaborated with the American Nurses Association to establish National Nurse Response teams as an essential component of the National Disaster Medical System. Carmona encouraged all nurses to be knowledgeable about emergency preparedness to educate their patients and deal with emergencies. He advocated expansion of nurses' sphere of influence to improve citizens' health and talked with the president about how to attract young men and women to nursing. His comments resonated with his nursing colleagues: "Nurses are an invaluable asset, an under-appreciated tool in our health armamentarium. From the bottom of my heart, I want to say thank you. We could not have a health system without nurses" (Wood, 2004).

Carmona returned to Arizona and public life there. In 2012, he lost a close race for Senator by less than three percentage points as a Democrat in a predominately Republican state (Duda, 2013). He continues to speak out on healthcare issues and remembers his nursing roots. In 2012, he delivered the keynote address for the Arizona Nurses Association Symposium, where he emphasized the importance of moving from a model of "sick care" to "health care" that focuses on prevention by reducing smoking and obesity (Moffett, 2012, p. 4). Carmona is a proponent of health literacy and preventive care in his work as president of the Canyon Ranch Institute, vice chairman of Canyon Ranch, and Distinguished Professor of Public Health at the University of Arizona. He advocates an integrative approach to "deal with issues of mind, body, and spirit to pursue optimal health and wellness" (Carmona, 2014, p. xv). On Canyon Ranch's 10th anniversary, he announced a partnership with The Ohio State University College of Nursing where he serves as Distinguished Professor of Health Promotion and Entrepreneurship. He and Dean Bernadette Melnyk, PhD, RN, are collaborating to establish innovative approaches in health literacy and prevention by beginning the first nurse-led Canyon Ranch Institute Life Enhancement Program in a low-income section of Columbus, Ohio (Carmona, 2013).

Carmona also weighed in during the recent Ebola crisis to promote nursing. When a nurses' union official at Texas Health Presbyterian Hospital in Dallas announced on CNN that protocols were not in place when the first patient diagnosed with Ebola was admitted there, he spoke up: "We have the nurses telling us they're unprepared.... I know that nurses are often the barometer of how hospitals function, because they're at the patient's bedside 7/24. So, we need to listen and take appropriate action" (Carruthers, 2014). He also took the opportunity to promote emergency preparedness at all times:

> *Every hospital, every doctor, every nurse has to understand the basic premises around all hazards preparedness, including these bioagents. People need...clear messaging that will give them information, but not inflame the situation—that will allow them to understand how they can best protect their families and their communities. Doctors, nurses, health professionals need that same information. (Carruthers, 2014)*

Richard Carmona has been a successful husband, father of four (one of whom is a nurse), soldier, nurse, physician, trauma surgeon, surgeon general, healthcare leader, author, and public safety official who has received numerous awards and honors. He has taken courageous and sometimes unpopular stands to promote population health and safety. His remarkable achievements are extraordinary for a street kid who had a vision and the determination to attain it.

His ultimate message for his colleagues in nursing and medicine resulted from his visit as surgeon general to the University of Pennsylvania Schools of Nursing and Medicine in 2004. The deans of both schools focused on partnership. According to Rich,

> *this is not a competition; we work together. So they have combined grand rounds, combined continuing education seminars and such. I think that is wonderful. That is the kind of esprit de corps we need to engender so that we are seen as a team. We work together. Our roles are complementary. (Mattson, 2005, p. 15)*

Richard Carmona continues to advance the health and safety of the American people as well as promoting the health professions he loves. His story isn't over and the next chapter has yet to be written. One thing is certain: It definitely won't be dull!

Implications for Nurse Leaders Today and in the Future
Courage

Merriam-Webster Dictionary defines courage as "the ability to do something that you know is difficult or dangerous" (Courage, n.d.). Richard

Carmona displayed courage in war and in his role as deputy sheriff, but those weren't the only times (Mattson, 2005). It took courage to speak out publically and before Congress in opposition to the administration that appointed him surgeon general about politicizing the office (Harris, 2007). It also took courage to support nurses during the Ebola crisis (Carruthers, 2014). Florence Nightingale also displayed courage in war and peace. She traveled to the Crimea to care for grievously wounded soldiers in appalling conditions. Before that, she volunteered to nurse patients at Middlesex Hospital during a cholera epidemic even though she wasn't employed there (Cook, 1913a). Those instances of courage marked the beginning of Nightingale's nursing career and the subsequent evolution of nursing.

Today's nurse leaders also face numerous challenges and must have the courage to confront them. When the Honor Society of Nursing, Sigma Theta Tau, was founded in 1922, it was based on three values: "Love, courage, and honor" (Hawkins & Morse, 2014, p. 263). Love has been replaced with caring and honor with ethical principles. Courage is not generally a topic in nursing literature and theory, but the concept is still important to nursing practice.

Nurses' participation in codes and emergencies is an expectation in clinical practice that is one manifestation of courage. It requires a calm, professional approach that ensures safe patient care. Nurse leaders realize that the stress these situations can cause to staff nurses often manifests itself after the crisis. They must advocate for debriefing and emotional support as an expectation every time. Although emergency care is a learned response, other examples of courage by nurses and nurse leaders are not. Risk-taking to advocate for patients is necessary, but not always rewarded. Courage requires moral strength to challenge threats of retaliation by others when patient care is compromised by unethical practice. It may be easier to be a code team member than to face a physician and challenge an inappropriate order or contact the Ethics Committee when a patient and family are not on the same page about palliative care. Often, the nurse leader is the go-to person when staff members are unsure how to approach a difficult physician, administrator, colleague, or family member.

It is imperative that nurse leaders model risk-taking actions, reinforce duty and responsibility, mentor others to practice courageously, and advocate for patients. They approach such situations with integrity and confidence and take action in difficult circumstances while keeping the patient at the center of care. Courageous actions like these aren't easy, but they are essential for patient safety and an opportunity to develop the courage of other nurses. "Courage makes a strong nurse confident enough to provide effective patient care essential for efficacy and excellence" (Hawkins & Morse, 2014, p. 269). With this in mind, nurse leaders must act courageously and guide others to do the same.

— *19* —

Eugene Sawicki
Priest and Nurse

(November 7, 1939–)

Eugene's Story

Eugene Sawicki didn't set out to become a doctorally prepared nurse. It just happened along the way, and his nursing skills have been invaluable to him ever since. Sawicki always wanted to be a Catholic priest and went to seminary after graduation from high school. He spent six years there, but his inquisitive nature wasn't welcomed. At that time, his vows expired and the faculty recommended that he leave the seminary and pursue some life experiences. He had completed four years of college by then, but had no degree (E. Sawicki, personal communication, August 15, 2015).

Sawicki was 24 when he left the seminary. He took some graduate medieval philosophy courses at Fordham University, but left without completing a degree. Then, he decided to take the advice of his seminary professors and gain life experiences by joining the Army in 1963 where he served with the U.S. Military Police in Germany for two years. After returning home, he taught in Harlem for the Irish Christian Brothers and Sisters of Mercy. The Sisters of Mercy introduced him to Mercy College where he would earn the first of his eight degrees (E. Sawicki, personal communication, August 15, 2015).

He still was passionate about the priesthood, but the Church wasn't ready for his direct, "tell it like it is" style. Since the priesthood was out of reach, he sought other employment that would change his life and provide opportunities that furthered his education. He joined the New York City Fire Department (FDNY) as a firefighter and stayed there 27 years in the Division of Fire Communications, earning more than 11 commendations. The FDNY 48 hours on/24 hours off schedule suited Sawicki well. He enrolled in school, attending all day and working in the FDNY at night for two days, before his day off. He loved his job and his studies. He also had the distinction of being the first male student at Mercy College. When he graduated with a Bachelor in Psychology degree in 1970, Sawicki was one of only four men in the graduating class. His pride in his first academic degree is evident as he still wears his ring from Mercy (Stasi, 1995; MercyCollege, 2010). Student loans and a flexible schedule (for someone who didn't require much sleep) led to more degrees. These included a Master's in Counseling Psychology from Manhattan College and a Master's in Theology from Woodstock College (MercyCollege, 1992).

The FDNY also led Sawicki to nursing. Hunter College's Bellevue School of Nursing offered a BSN for firefighters and teachers and he took advantage of it (Sawicki, 2015). Nursing fascinated him, particularly its emphasis on the whole person, not just the physical aspects of care. He saw the linkage between nursing and the priesthood—the physical and spiritual (Barnum, 2001). That belief was expressed in Florence Nightingale's view of nursing that "nursing was a Sacred Calling, only to be followed by those who felt the vocation, and only followed to good purpose by those who pursued it as the service of God through the highest kind of service to man" (Cook, 1913b, p. 269). Although Eugene Sawicki was not yet a priest, he embraced Nightingale's view of the nursing profession.

He also gained more nursing skills and knowledge by obtaining a Master's in Nursing Education and a Master's of Education in Gerontology from Columbia. After that, Sawicki wanted to pursue a nursing doctorate from Teachers College at Columbia University. He met the Dean wearing a propeller hat and managed to get admitted to the program anyway. In 1986, he submitted his dissertation topic "What do Nursing Deans Do?" where he humorously compared ordinary and excellent nursing deans. His faculty committee enjoyed reading his results and he became a Doctor of Nursing Education (Sawicki, 2015; MercyCollege, 1992).

Then, he heard that a Lithuanian Catholic church, Our Lady of Vilnius, by the Holland Tunnel needed a priest. When he heard that he would have to go to Rome and study canon law, he protested. Then, he went anyway for two years. After graduating with a Licentiate of Canon Law from the Pontifical Gregorian University in Rome, he finally had an opportunity for ordination (MercyCollege, 1992; Stasi, 1995). In 1987, he was ordained as a deacon and assigned to a Haitian church in Brooklyn. He also returned to work at the FDNY. When a church official from Rome called to check on him, the priest at the church mentioned that Deacon Sawicki had baptized 27 people the day before. Soon after, he was finally ordained as a priest by Bishop Paul Baltakis, OFM, on December 6, 1986, at St. Patrick's Cathedral (Bulvičius, 2000). At 47, Father Eugene Sawicki achieved the goal he had sought for over 20 years.

Luckily, it was his day off from the FDNY because he still worked there and would for eight more years. He added in some other activities as well. He was an advisory board member of Mercy's Therapeutic Recreation Program and began teaching at Mercy as an adjunct professor in 1982. Students loved his humor, compassion, knowledge, and his unique teaching style. After his ordination, Father Eugene served as a military chaplain in the New York State Guard with a rank of lieutenant colonel and later was appointed by Cardinal O'Connor to the New York State Interdiocesan Appellate Court as a judge over marriage cases (MercyCollege, 1992, 2010).

When Father Eugene's Lithuanian and Polish ancestry landed him at Our Lady of Vilnius, he didn't speak or write Lithuanian, which didn't prove to be an obstacle. His warm, caring personality and humor endeared him to his diverse parishioners. His Masses included practical messages along with the Gospel and his Sunday Masses were in Lithuanian as he learned the language (Nobody's Wife, 2006; Anderson, 2006). Father Eugene retired from the FDNY in 1995 after eight years at Our Lady of Vilnius. During that time, he worked nights in the Central Park Manhattan Fire Command Station and spent his days as a priest, using his nursing assessment skills in both roles (Stasi, 1995).

After his retirement from the FDNY, Father Eugene combined the priesthood and nursing in his daily activities. Firehouse memorabilia and a scanner in his living quarters demonstrated his pride in the FDNY. When not wearing a clerical collar, he usually wore an FDNY t-shirt. One parishioner had this to say of him:

The best of the FDNY had become a part of Father Eugene's outlook, manifesting itself in the heart and humor that expressed itself in casual exchanges, in homilies and in compassion for the failings of the average man and woman. We are proud to have a pastor that had been numbered among New York's Bravest and happy to benefit from every good thing that he carried from that experience into the priesthood. (Nobody's Wife, 2007)

The parishioners knew that he was a nurse and felt comfortable talking with him about physical, as well as spiritual, issues. He automatically assessed their needs and added a spiritual element to nursing, particularly when assisting the dying. His philosophical and theological education showed him that there are seven levels of personality to address. They are theological (thoughts of God), philosophical (questions about existence), psychological (seeing people as individuals), sociological (seeing individuals as part of a group), economic (practical considerations), aesthetic (looking at beauty), and physical (caring for the body). In his words, "nursing and the priesthood share many things. They both call for healing at the seven levels of personhood. You are constantly calling upon what you know; assessing, intervening, and calling on all your resources" (Barnum, 2001, p. 156).

He has published articles in theological and nursing publications and been a member of the Sigma Theta Tau nursing honor society. In June 1990, he was selected to represent the Archdiocese of New York and spoke at the United Nations for the XIV International Congress for Catholic Nurses and Health-Care Workers. Father Eugene's presentation, "Ethics and Decision-Making in a Changing World," shared his unique perspective about the need for professional nurses to be 'synthetic thinkers' who analyze findings and apply them at all levels of practice in ethical decision-making rather than just attending an ethics course. His international audience loved it (MercyCollege, 1992; Sawicki, 2015).

His approach to both professions was tested in the aftermath of September 11, 2001, after the bombing of the World Trade Center. Father Eugene spent nights at Ground Zero for months assisted by three Lutheran women deacons. Together, they ministered to firefighters, police, and residents who needed physical and emotional support. His skills in crisis intervention and nursing helped his fellow New Yorkers deal with a catastrophic situation. They avoided publicity and quietly went about their business. That was Father Eugene's style. In discussing this period, he said that the

Therapeutic Recreation Program at Mercy College was "helpful in those nights" (Sawicki, 2015), but didn't promote himself in any way. What was important to Father Eugene was that people who needed help received it.

After 20 years at Our Lady of Vilnius, Father Eugene faced another crisis, but this one involved the Catholic Church itself. In the winter of 2004, some of the trusses holding up the church roof cracked and the Archdiocese put a three-story scaffolding in the sanctuary to support the ceiling. Repairs were never made and a new ceiling was never installed even though the problem was reported. Father Eugene was unable to use the sanctuary for services, weddings, or funerals. All functions occurred in the basement (Anderson, 2006).

On July 31, 2006, he was summoned to a meeting with Cardinal Edward Egan, who informed him that the Church would be closed at a future date. The congregation began a five-year unsuccessful battle to save their church. On February 27, 2007, Father Eugene was informed by the Cardinal that he was locking the doors and that he should contact the Buildings Department to get his belongings: clothes, books, chalice. He dislikes publicity, but consented to an interview to support Our Lady of Vilnius and his congregation's spiritual health, saying,

> it's not only about me, and the treatment of a priest. It's about the parishioners. The old people who used to come here every day to play cards and cook now have nowhere to go. There's nowhere to celebrate the liturgy. They're outside in the cold. That's not right. This is a place where people come to be in the presence of God. Good liturgy is good theater, and good theater is good therapy. St. Vilnius raises the hearts and minds to God. (Stasi, 2007).

Today, the Church is gone. The Cardinal is gone. The parishioners have gone elsewhere. Rev. Dr. Eugene Sawicki—priest and nurse—remains. He says Mass in other parishes, performs weddings and funerals, and uses his nursing skills as he interacts with others. He demonstrates the importance of critical thinking and the unity of science and spirituality. In his words: "Has nursing helped me be a better priest? Of course it has, by making me attentive to the practical in living. Once a nurse, always a nurse; it's a mark on the soul" (Barnum, 2001, pp. 154–155).

In the words of St. Augustine on serving those in need: "What does love look like? It has the hands to help others. It has the feet to hasten to the poor and needy. It has eyes to see misery and want. It has the ears to hear the sighs and sorrows of men. That is what love looks like" (Carey, 2014). This is the legacy of Rev. Dr. Eugene Sawicki, priest and nurse.

Implications for Nurse Leaders Today and in the Future
Spirituality

Spirituality is a concept usually not addressed by nurse leaders today. Yet it is a vital aspect of patients' lives that impacts their response to care. Rev. Dr. Sawicki believes that spirituality and science are one (Sawicki, 2015). Nightingale believed that spirituality did not refer to a specific religion, but had a practical purpose. In her words:

> *The way to live with God is to live with Ideas—not merely to think about ideals, but to do and suffer for them. Those who have to work on men and women must above all things have their Spiritual Ideal, their purpose, ever present. The "mystical" state is the essence of common sense. (Cook, 1913b, p. 235)*

Keeping both of these beliefs in mind, today's nurse leaders must make spirituality essential to leadership and managing by role modeling and empowering others to explore the value of spirituality in practice. In this context, spirituality focuses on responsibility and accountability for nursing practice and the ability to question practice issues for the patient's benefit. Nurses must feel appreciated themselves to make patients feel respected and valued (Smith & Robinson, 2015).

Spirituality requires the nurse leader to enable staff empowerment by facilitating (Smith & Robinson, 2015):

1. *Consciousness* of the other person (patient)
2. *Connectivity* to appreciate relationships with the other person (patient)
3. *Criticality* involving positive testing of differences
4. *Commitment* to the person, purpose, and project
5. *Community* to provide a context for care that develops relationships and trust

6. *Character* to emphasize qualities that strengthen spirituality and are strengthened by spirituality (enable responsible action and leadership)

7. *Creativity* to take action that helps people feel recognized and valued

Based on these seven Cs, spirituality encompasses physical care and caring relationships as much as feelings or ideas. Today, when patient perceptions influence reimbursement and patients have multiple options where to receive care, spirituality must be at the center of organizational management, nursing leadership, and patient care. Today's nurse leaders must embrace this concept of spirituality themselves to instill it in their nurses. The unity of science and spirituality and its practical application to practice truly supports quality patient care and a positive patient experience.

$$\sim 20 \sim$$

Peter Buerhaus

Nursing Workforce Scholar

(May 10, 1954–)

Peter's Story

Peter Buerhaus was born in Zanesville, Ohio, where his father was a hospital administrator. His childhood was spent in Ohio and South Dakota as his father's career evolved. He learned how hospitals functioned and his first choice for his own career was to become a physician. Then, his sister became a nurse and her enthusiasm was infectious. A number of physician associates also pushed him to consider nursing (Murdock, 2006).

He realized that nursing was an opportunity to interact directly with patients, families, and the community. Nursing also focuses on prevention while physicians focus on disease pathology and treatment modalities. Both disciplines must demonstrate interprofessional collaboration for health care to succeed. Buerhaus enrolled in the BSN program at Minnesota State Mankato and enjoyed the opportunities it provided to learn the why as well as how of nursing practice. His classmates and professors stimulated his knowledge of his new profession. It was a thoroughly positive experience (Frederick, 2014). He didn't experience the gender discrimination that men faced in nursing in earlier times. When interviewed for an article about men in nursing in 2013, Buerhaus affirmed this: "People notice that when they come out of high school, there's no longer a negative stigma" (Gross, 2013).

After graduation in 1976, Buerhaus wanted to see the world. He planned to work until he could afford a flight to another country and to seek employment as a nurse wherever he traveled. It was a good plan, but life got in the way (Frederick, 2014). He met Lorraine, fell in love, and married. He spent the next few years as a hospital nurse. In his second position, Buerhaus was promoted to head nurse, but not in a positive context. The unit's previous head nurse had been in that position for years and was liked and respected by the staff. It was an impossible position for the newly appointed head nurse. He was concerned about the capricious nature of the decision and his inability to advocate for himself and the other staff nurses. He made a decision to return to school for a master's degree in health administration and found his future career direction there (Frederick, 2014).

Buerhaus entered the master's program at the University of Michigan and took a class in economics. His teacher stimulated his interest in the subject and he enrolled in a healthcare economics course. He found his passions— nursing and economics. At the time, most people in both professions didn't consider the relevance of the other one. Buerhaus began to analyze research results from well-planned economics studies and saw the significance of those results to nursing practice and policy. His excitement led him to education for advanced roles (Murdock, 2006; Frederick, 2014).

After graduation with his Master's in Nursing Health Services Administration in 1981, Buerhaus completed a Master's in Community Health Nursing from Wayne State University in 1983. For the next three years, he was assistant to the CEO of the University of Michigan Medical Center's seven teaching hospitals. From 1987 to 1990, he was assistant to the Vice Provost for Medical Affairs, the CEO of the Medical Center. Both positions enabled him to view hospitals and health care from a leadership perspective. During his seven years at the Medical Center, Buerhaus pursued his doctoral degree in healthcare economics at Wayne State (Vanderbilt University, Department of Health Policy, 2015).

Buerhaus was debating his dissertation topic when his wife read a newspaper article about a looming nursing shortage. Neither of them realized when she suggested the topic for his dissertation that it would be the foundation for his expertise on nursing workforce issues (Murdock,

2006). He was awarded his PhD in 1990 and joined the University of Iowa faculty. There he created and taught public policy-making and health care and nursing economics and began his academic career (Hall & Manley, 2003). Then, he received a postdoctoral faculty fellowship in healthcare finance from the Robert Wood Johnson Foundation at the Johns Hopkins University. In 1992, he was employed at the Harvard School of Public Health as Assistant Professor of Health Policy and Management (Vanderbilt University, Department of Health Policy, 2015).

During his eight years there, Buerhaus's reputation as a nurse economist and researcher grew nationally and Vanderbilt University recruited him in 2000 as Senior Associate Dean for Research. This position evolved into multiple roles there, including "the Valere Potter Distinguished Professor of Nursing at Vanderbilt University School of Nursing, Director of the Center for Interdisciplinary Health Workforce Studies, and Professor in the Department of Health Policy in the Institute for Medicine and Public Health at Vanderbilt University Medical Center" (Vanderbilt University, Department of Health Policy, 2015).

Peter Buerhaus has received numerous awards and recognition as the foremost nurse–economist in the country and was named the Chair of the National Health Care Workforce Commission in 2010. The Commission is a resource for government entities that is responsible for evaluating education and training, identifying barriers and ways to resolve them, and encouraging innovations to meet population needs. His expertise in nursing workforce economics and his positive approach to seek solutions to healthcare workforce needs made him a logical choice for this role (Vanderbilt University, Department of Health Policy, 2015).

His research on healthcare workforce issues is prolific and he is the recognized authority on nursing shortage/employment trends, contributions of nurses to quality of care using nurse-sensitive indicators, and the contributions of nurse practitioners in primary care delivery. Dr. Buerhaus has published over 100 articles in peer-reviewed journals. Five of these publications are considered 'classics' by AHRQ (the Agency for Healthcare Research and Quality) and others are among the most frequently accessed articles in the journal *Health Affairs* (Vanderbilt University, Department of Health Policy, 2015). His literary accomplishments mirror those of another nurse leader: Florence Nightingale, whose publications on sanitation in India were widely disseminated and reflected her in-depth research on the topic (Cook, 1913b). Buerhaus's impressive number of publications and research studies have been recognized by healthcare leaders and policy makers as integral to value-driven nursing care in the climate of healthcare reform. He advocates that nurses have numerous opportunities to prove their value by "nursing economic accountability" (Douglas & Kerfoot, 2011, p. 169).

In the spring of 2015, Peter Buerhaus joined Montana State University to teach undergraduate and graduate nursing courses. He looked forward to living in the area and wanted to participate in research about the rural healthcare workforce and the health of Native Americans. It was another example of Peter Buerhaus seeking challenges and new learning experiences professionally and personally (MSU, 2014). For Peter and Lorraine, it will be an exciting adventure.

Buerhaus's accomplishments are remarkable and his contributions to the fields of nursing and economics continue. He is popular and respected by his colleagues and the officials and thought leaders he interacts with on a daily basis. Most of all, he remains grounded as a nurse. He is a true advocate for direct care nurses and passionate about fostering their success. In his own words: "When interacting with other nurses, never forget that the nursing profession is the greatest of all professions. Every nurse deserves your respect" (Murdock, 2006).

One thing is clear, his fellow nurses should be proud to have Peter Buerhaus represent the nursing profession now and in the future. He does it well and Nightingale would be gratified that her vision of professional nursing is thriving and evolving in the 21st century!

Implications for Nurse Leaders Today and in the Future
Nursing Economic Accountability

Peter Buerhaus recognizes that nurses are crucial to the success or failure of their organizations. Nurses and their organizations must be linked to each other. Nightingale knew this in the 1860s when she developed plans for ideal hospitals and the trained nurses to staff them. According to her biographer, "the improvement of buildings and of nursing went on concurrently and Miss Nightingale used her influence in each department to improve the other" (Cook, 1913b, pp. 185–186).

Healthcare reform has brought a new language along with a focus on value-driven care that emphasizes clinical outcomes and patient perceptions. Value-based purchasing (VBP) bases reimbursement on publically reported clinical outcomes and HCAHPS scores about patient perceptions compared to peer group benchmarks. Improved performance is rewarded financially. Hospitals with poor outcomes and/or low HCAHPS scores are penalized by reduced Medicare reimbursement resulting in potentially significant revenue reductions (Volland, 2014).

Today's nurse leaders have enormous responsibility to ensure that nurses practice economic accountability in their daily activities to obtain the best possible return on value-based purchasing and, most of all, to demonstrate the power of nurses within their facilities. Nursing units are usually considered cost, rather than revenue, centers and healthcare reform is an exciting opportunity for nurses to affect their hospital's bottom line. Nurses influence clinical process of care outcomes including nurse-sensitive indicators related to healthcare-associated infections (Medicare.gov, 2014). They also greatly effect patients' perception of care. Their technical and interpersonal skills are the most effective tactics in hospital reimbursement through VBP (Volland, 2014)

Unfortunately, many nurses fail to see how important they are to their organizations and many organizations don't recognize nurses' contributions. For both to thrive, they must understand each other. Nurse leaders must educate nurses about healthcare financing, economic incentives for providers, and how they can use this knowledge in their practice. Cost reduction is not always an option for nurses, but reducing waste and increasing efficiency are options. Increasing efficiency and effectiveness requires practicing with economic accountability. Nurse leaders must promote innovations and ideas that will enable nurses to work smarter, not harder. Their nurses must see themselves as visionaries who improve their practice and achieve clinical process of care outcomes and improved patient perceptions of care (Douglas & Kerfoot, 2011).

Nurse leaders are responsible for marketing their nurses' accomplishments in practicing economic accountability to the administration and particularly the CFO and finance department. They need to know the positive impact the nurses have on the bottom line on an ongoing basis. This is imperative to ensure that nurse staffing reflects nursing's importance and integration within the organization and the patients it serves. Today's dynamic and fluctuating healthcare environment is an opportunity for the nursing profession to evolve by practicing "with greater economic accountability to fully realize the profession's potential" (Douglas & Kerfoot, 2011, p. 172). Today's nurse leaders need to join Peter Buerhaus in showing how nurses contribute to their organizations and society to reduce waste and costs and improve patient satisfaction and access to care. Nursing is the most respected profession and nursing leaders are in a unique position to demonstrate the value of nurses and play a leadership role in the future of health care, not just for their organizations, but for the future of their profession. It's a challenge that American nurse leaders must accept to carry on Nightingale's legacy.

Epilogue

Study the past if you would define the future.

—Confucius

You have read the stories of 20 representative American nurse leaders—men, women, African American, white, Hispanic, and Native American from Nightingale's time to today. Each of their lives has implications for the nurse leaders of today and tomorrow. The evolution of American nurse leaders continues to demonstrate that Nightingale's legacy is alive and well. Now, the challenge for significant nurse leaders of the 21st century is to leverage these lessons and advance the profession of nursing into an exciting and challenging future.

Remembering Nightingale's accomplishments in the Crimea, it is appropriate to close this book with the words of a nurse from the battlefields of another war—Civil War nurse and poet Walt Whitman (Whitman 2015):

The Wound Dresser

1

An old man bending I come among new faces,
Years looking backward resuming in answer to children,
Come tell us old man, as from young men and maidens that love me,
(Arous'd and angry, I'd thought to beat the alarum, and urge relentless war,
But soon my fingers failed me, my face droop'd and I resign'd myself,
To sit by the wounded and soothe them, or silently watch the dead;)
Years hence of these scenes, of these furious passions, these chances,
Of unsurpass'd heroes (was one side so brave? The other was equally brave;)
Now be witness again, paint the mightiest armies of earth,
Of those armies so rapid so wondrous what saw you to tell us?
What stays with you latest and deepest? Of curious panics,
Of hard-fought engagements or sieges tremendous what deepest remains?

2

O maidens and young men I love and that love me,
What you ask of my days those the strangest and sudden your talking recalls,
Soldier alert I arrive after a long march cover'd with sweat and dust,
In the nick of time I come, plunge in the fight, loudly shout in the rush of
     successful charge,
Enter the captur'd works—yet lo, like a swift running river they fade,
Pass and are gone they fade—I dwell not on soldiers' perils or soldiers' joys,
(Both I remember well—many of the hardships, few the joys, yet I was content.)
But in silence, in dreams' projections,
While the world of gain and appearance and mirth goes on,
So soon what is over forgotten, and waves wash the imprints off the sand,
With hinged knees returning I enter the doors, (while for you up there,
Whoever you are, follow without noise and be of strong heart.)
Bearing the bandages, water and sponge,
Straight and swift to my wounded I go,
Where they lie on the ground after the battle brought in,
Where their priceless blood reddens the grass, the ground,
Or to the rows of the hospital tent, or under the roof'd hospital,
To the long rows of cots up and down each side I return,
To each and all one after another I draw near, not one do I miss,
An attendant follows holding a tray, he carries a refuse pail,
Soon to be fill'd with clotted rags and blood, emptied, and fill'd again.
I onward go, I stop,
With hinged knees and steady hand to dress wounds,
I am firm with each, the pangs are sharp yet unavoidable,

One turns to me his appealing eyes—poor boy! I never knew you,
Yet I think I could not refuse this moment to die for you, if that would save you.

3

On, on I go, (open doors of time! open hospital doors!)
The crush'd head I dress, (poor crazed hand tear not the bandage away,)
The neck of the cavalry-man with the bullet through and through I examine,
Hard the breathing rattles, quite glazed already the eye, yet life struggles hard,
(Come sweet death! be persuaded O beautiful death!
In mercy come quickly.)
From the stump of the arm, the amputated hand,
I undo the clotted lint, remove the slough, wash off the matter and blood,
Back on his pillow the soldier bends with curv'd neck and side falling head,
His eyes are closed, his face is pale, he dares not look on the bloody stump,
And has not yet look'd on it.
I dress a wound in the side, deep, deep,
But a day or two more, for see the frame all wasted and sinking,
And the yellow-blue countenance see.
I dress the perforated shoulder, the foot with the bullet-wound,
Cleanse the one with a gnawing and putrid gangrene, so sickening, so offensive,
While the attendant stands behind aside me holding the tray and pail.
I am faithful, I do not give out,
The fractur'd thigh, the knee, the would in the abdomen,
These and more I dress with impassive hand (yet deep in my breast a fire, a
    burning flame.)

4

Thus in silence in dreams' projections,
Returning, resuming, I thread my way through the hospitals,
The hurt and wounded I pacify with soothing hand,
I sit by the restless all the dark night, some are so young,
Some suffer so much, I recall the experience sweet and sad,
(Many a soldier's loving arms about this neck have cross'd and rested,
Many a soldier's kiss dwells on these bearded lips.)

Afterword

Nightingale Legacy Leaders and Nurse Leadership Competencies

Now you have come to the end of the book and have a choice to make. You can close the book, put it on a shelf in your bookcase, and forget about it. Or, you can use the following table—which maps characteristics of the nurse leaders profiled in these pages to the competencies of ANA's leadership professional performance standard (ANA 2015b, p. 75)—to let its lessons guide your practice to benefit patients, interprofessional colleagues, fellow nurses, and yourself. (A competency in the context of nursing is the expected and measurable level of performance that integrates knowledge, skills, abilities, and judgment and is based on established knowledge and expectations of nursing practice [ANA, 2015b; p. 44].) You could also use it to guide you in further study of these profiles: most of these nurses would map to at least several of these competencies. The choice is yours!

TABLE 1 **Nightingale Legacy Nurse Leaders and the Standard of Professional Nursing Practice for Leadership**

Standard 11. Leadership: The registered nurse leads within the professional practice setting and the profession.

Competency	Nightingale legacy nurse leaders who demonstrated this competency	Implications for current nurse leaders
Contributes to the establishment of an environment that supports and maintains respect, trust, and dignity.	**Ethical Practice** Isabel Hampton Robb **Spirituality** Eugene Sawicki	Spirituality and ethical practice are cornerstones in establishing an environment that is respectful and trustworthy for patients and colleagues. All nurse leaders must role-model the provisions of the Code of Ethics for Nurses in their daily practice. They must empower staff nurses to question practice issues for their patients' benefit and keep spirituality at the center of organizational management, nursing leadership and patient care.
Encourages innovation in practice and role performance to attain personal and professional plans, goals, and visions.	**Caring and Culture** Madeleine Leininger **Political Savvy** Mary Breckinridge	Practice innovations require nurturing and political savvy about the organizational climate to succeed. Cultural changes start with a vision and a desire for goal achievement that improves quality care. Nurse leaders are in a unique position to challenge the status quo and guide innovations by developing political savvy and social intelligence to gain support for their vision.
Communicates to manage change and address conflict.	**Courage** Richard Carmona **Dealing with Difficult People** Mabel Keaton Staupers	Conflict is inevitable in health care and in life. Nurse leaders must project professionalism and respect when negotiating with challenging people to effect positive change. They must have the courage to confront issues while focusing on resolution and mentor others to do the same.
Mentors colleagues for the advancement of nursing practice and the profession to enhance safe, quality health care.	**Promoting Education** Mary Adelaide Nutting **Patient-Centered Care** Virginia Henderson	Nurse leaders must promote education for themselves and other nurses to advance nursing practice and the profession. They must be knowledgeable about undergraduate and graduate education opportunities to guide colleagues into establishing personal education pathways. They also must advocate patient-centered care as a key component in both patient and nurse satisfaction and safe, quality health care.
Retains . accountability for delegated nursing care.	**The Importance of Delegation** Clara Barton	Nurse leaders understand that delegation—transferring to another the responsibility for a task while retaining accountability for the outcome—is essential to achieve desired results. Their personal leadership style, education, and confidence in delegation to the correct individual(s) enhance communication effectiveness, develop positive working relationships, and increase trust. Effective delegation requires experience and confidence that grows with practice. Nurse leaders develop others to succeed when they delegate appropriately, resulting in positive benefits to the delegate, the patients, the unit, and the organization.

Competency	Nightingale legacy nurse leaders who demonstrated this competency	Implications for current nurse leaders
Contributes to the evolution of the profession through participation in professional organizations.	**Legislative Advocacy** Lavinia Lloyd Dock **Change Agent** Estelle Riddle Osborne	Nurse leaders must participate in professional organizations to advance the profession. They can accomplish this in two ways. The first is to ensure that laws regulating nursing practice meet current and future standards for the profession. The second is to lead change in their organizations and community by trying new approaches and keeping pace with best practices. Their commitment to growth enables them to influence their colleagues, and pursue change with knowledge and positive communication skills.
Influences policy to promote health.	**Nursing Economic Accountability** Peter Buerhaus **Importance of Statistical Analysis** Margaret Sanger	Nurse leaders must educate nurses about healthcare financing, economic incentives for providers, and how they can use this knowledge in their practice. Cost reduction is not always an option. Reducing waste and increasing efficiency and effectiveness require practicing with economic accountability. Nurse leaders must market their nurses' accomplishments in practicing economic accountability to the administration and particularly the CFO and finance department. They also use multiple data sources and statistical information as evidence to influence policy to promote health and quality patient care.
Influences decision-making bodies to improve the professional practice environment and healthcare consumer outcomes.*	**Health Promotion** Annie Warburton Goodrich **Importance of Assessment** Susie Walking Bear Yellowtail	Nurse leaders influence decision-making bodies to improve healthcare consumer outcomes by their skills in using assessment data to improve nursing practice at the unit and service line levels and nursing outcomes at the organizational level. They use these resources in consultation with other leaders to achieve results that enhance nursing practice. Nurse leaders also focus beyond the walls of the facility when coordinating patient care. Promoting health across the continuum is a goal in today's complex healthcare system. Nurse leaders must ensure that staff nurses are able to spend time with patients and families helping them achieve goals for wellness and encouraging their participation in care. Nurse leaders must be knowledgeable about community resources available for patients to prevent readmissions and ensure their safety.
Enhances the effectiveness of the interprofessional team.*	**Living Cultural Diversity** Lillian Wald	Nurse leaders realize the importance of diversity and know that race and ethnic background influence health outcomes. Nurse leaders must educate themselves and other health team members about health practices of the population in their service areas—racial, ethnic, religious, sexual, and cultural. They must promote ongoing discussion with members of these communities and ensure advocacy for these practices in the healthcare environment. They must also seek diversity in hiring to reflect population demographics.
Promotes advanced practice nursing and role development by interpreting its role for healthcare consumers and policy makers.*	**Innovation** Luther Christman **Contribute to Professional Literature** Mary Elizabeth Carnegie	Nurse leaders must use innovative approaches in their roles to advance nursing in their facilities and as a profession. Nurses are capable of being innovators and change agents by creating unit changes that can result in improvements in patient care and organizational efficiency and effectiveness. Nurse leaders must encourage out-of-the-box thinking and provide nurses with the resources they need to encourage innovative solutions to nursing and healthcare problems. Nurse leaders must add to the profession's body of knowledge by sharing their own knowledge and expertise. Although research articles are always welcome, a well-written perspective about a clinical topic will be valuable to readers who are seeking information that they can use in their practice.

(Continued)

Competency	Nightingale legacy nurse leaders who demonstrated this competency	Implications for current nurse leaders
Models expert practice to interprofessional team members and healthcare consumers.*	**Excellence in Care Delivery** Mary Eliza Mahoney	The most important aspect of nurse leadership is ensuring quality patient care. Basic nursing care has never been more important and must be a priority. Evidence-based strategies create an environment for this and nurse leaders must play a significant role in achieving this priority. Nurse leaders must formulate a business case for nurse staffing that improves clinical quality and safety for patients. They must also increase nurses' efficiency and effectiveness by using Lean techniques to reduce time wasters that keep nurses from patient care. Shared decision-making engages staff nurses to champion issues that will enhance patient care delivery.
Mentors colleagues in the acquisition of clinical knowledge, skills, abilities, and judgment.*	**Global Collaboration** Linda Richards	Nurse leaders have an obligation to encourage and support nurses in attaining additional formal education to benefit the profession and patients. Nursing and patient care are global and nurse leaders have opportunities to share information with colleagues in distant lands. Although regional issues may differ, there are common priorities that nurse leaders can address globally to impact practice settings and meet current and future challenges in nursing and health care internationally. It is the responsibility of nurse leaders to continue international collaboration for the benefit of nurses and patients worldwide.

* Additional competencies for the APRN and the graduate-level prepared registered nurse.

Source: ANA, 2015b, p. 75

References

Altman, M., & Rosa, W. (2015). Redefining "time" to meet nursing's evolving demands. *Nursing Management, 46*(5), 46–50.

American Association for the History of Nursing. (c. 2007a). *AAHN research awards.* Retrieved July 3, 2015, from https://www.aahn.org/awards.html

American Association for the History of Nursing. (c. 2007b). *Lavinia Lloyd Dock 1858–1956.* Retrieved July 3, 2015, from https://www.aahn.org/gravesites/dock.html

American Nurses Association. (2012). *Frequently asked questions—Roles of state boards of nursing: Licensure, regulation and complaint investigation.* Retrieved July 3, 2015, from http://nursingworld.org/MainMenuCategories/Tools/State-Boards-of-Nursing-FAQ.pdf

American Nurses Association. (2015a). *Code of ethics for nurses with interpretive statements.* Washington, DC: Nursesbooks.org.

American Nurses Association. (2015b). *Nursing: Scope & standards of practice* (3rd ed.). Silver Spring, MD: Nursesbooks.org.

American Nurses Association. (2015c). *Susie Walking Bear Yellowtail (1903–1981) 2002 inductee.* Retrieved August 10, 2015, from http://www.nursingworld.org/SusieWalkingBearYellowtail

American Society of Registered Nurses. (2007, November 1). Big heart. *The Chronicle of Nursing.* Retrieved August 10, 2015, from http://www.asrn.org/journal-chronicle-nursing/205-big-heart.html

Anderson, L. (2006, August 23–29). Lady of Vilnius and 'Pretzels' and 'Provolone' may lose home. *The Villager, 76*(14). Retrieved August 30, 2015, from http://thevillager.com/villager_173/ladyofvilnius.html

Arizona Latin-American Medical Association. (c. 2014). *ALMA scholarship recipients*. Retrieved August 30, 2015, from http://www.almahealthcare.com/alma-2014-scholarship-recipients/

Barnum, B. S. (2001). Interview with Eugene Sawicki, RN, EdD, MDiv, JCL: When the nurse is a priest. In H. R. Feldman (Ed.), *Nursing Leaders Speak Out: Issues and Opinions* (pp. 151–158). New York, NY: Springer Publishing Company.

Barton, C. (1907). *The story of my childhood*. New York, NY: Baker & Taylor.

Block, I. (1969). *Neighbor to the world: The story of Lillian Wald*. New York, NY: Thomas Y. Crowell Company.

Bowers, P., & Ferron, L. (2014). Confronting conflict with higher-ups. *American Nurse Today, 9*(1), 52, 62.

Brandon, R., & Seldman, M. (2004). *Survival of the savvy: High integrity political tactics for career and company success*. New York, NY: Free Press.

Breckinridge, M. (1952). *Wide neighborhoods: A story of the Frontier Nursing Service*. Louisville, KY: The University Press of Kentucky.

Brown-Pryor, E. (1987). *Clara Barton, professional angel*. Philadelphia, PA: University of Pennsylvania Press.

Bulviẍius, D. (2000). 90 years for God & country [Weblog]. Retrieved September 4, 2015, from https://drive.google.com/file/d/0B89eTC_1ZePMMjdlN2M1NjItN2M5ZS00YTQ3LWEzNDctNDZhNzE4MjBmM2Zj/view?usp=drive_web&pli=1

Cameron, M. E., McIsaac, I., Dock, L. L., Nutting, A., & Robb, I. H. (1910). Memorial sketches of Isabel Adams Hampton Robb. *American Journal of Nursing, 11*(1), 9–43. Available from http://journals.lww.com/ajnonline/toc/1910/10000

Campbell, J. Y. (2012). In search of respect and equality: Life incidents of slave and free women in North American and European colonies. Self-published.

Carey, J. (2014). 15 St. Augustine quotes helped shape modern Christian thought. *Relevant*. Retrieved September 5, 2015, from http://www.relevantmagazine.com/god/15-augustine-quotes-helped-shape-modern-christian-thought

Carmona, R. (2013). Canyon Ranch Institute—Celebrating a decade of dedication to health & wellness. Canyon Ranch—The power of possibility. Retrieved August 30, 2015, from http://www.canyonranch.com/connection/winter-2013/cri-10th-anniversary

Carmona, R. (2014). *30 days to a better brain*. New York, NY: Atria Books.

Carnegie, M. E. (1991). *The path we tread: Blacks in nursing 1854–1990* (2nd ed.). New York, NY: National League for Nursing Press.

Carruthers, W. (2014, October 15). Former Surgeon General Carmona: Listen to nurses on Ebola. *Newsmax*. Retrieved August 30, 2015, from http://www.newsmax.com/Newsfront/Ebola-Texas-Nurses-healthcare/2014/10/15/id/600884/

Childs, B. (2012). Masters in nursing: Susie Walking Bear Yellowtail. Retrieved August 10, 2015 from http://nursinglicensemap.com/masters-in-nursing-susie-walking-bear-yellowtail/

Christman, L. P. (2011). Luther P. Christman Papers. Rush University Medical Center Archives. Chicago, IL. Retrieved August 22, 2015, from http://rushu.libguides.com/ld.php?content_id=8365378

Christman, L. P. (2015). Luther P. Christman Papers. Eskind Biomedical Library Special Collections. Nashville, TN. Retrieved August 22, 2015, from http://www.mc.vanderbilt.edu/diglib/se_diglib/archColl/16.html (link no longer active)

Cook, E. (1913a). *The life of Florence Nightingale* (Vol. 1). London, England: Macmillan.

Cook, E. (1913b). *The life of Florence Nightingale* (Vol. 2). London, England: Macmillan.

Courage. (n.d.). In *Merriam-Webster online*. Retrieved August 30, 2015, from http://www.merriam-webster.com/dictionary/courage

Darraj, S. M. (2005). *Mary Eliza Mahoney and the legacy of African-American nurses.* New York, NY: Chelsea House Publishers.

Davis, A. (1999). *Early black American leaders in nursing: Architects for integration and equality.* Sudbury, MA: Jones & Bartlett Publishers.

Department of Health and Human Services. (2006). *The health consequences of involuntary exposure to tobacco smoke: A report of the surgeon general.* Atlanta, GA: Centers for Disease Control. Retrieved August 30, 2015, from http://www.ncbi.nlm.nih.gov/books/NBK44324/pdf/Bookshelf_NBK44324.pdf

Dock, L. L. (1900). What we may expect from the law. *American Journal of Nursing, 1*(1), 8–12.

Dock, L. L., & Stewart, I. M. (1938). *A short history of nursing* (4th ed.). New York, NY: G. P. Putnam's Sons.

Douglas, E. T. (1975). *Margaret Sanger: Pioneer of the future.* Garrett Park, MD: Garrett Park Press.

Dossey, B. M. (2000). *Florence-Nightingale: Mystic, visionary, healer.* Springhouse, PA: Springhouse Corporation.

Douglas, K., & Kerfoot, K. (2011). Conversation with Peter Buerhaus. *Nursing Economic$, 29*(4), 169–182.

Draper, E. A. (1902). Isabel Hampton Robb. *American Journal of Nursing, 2*(4), 243–245. Retrieved July 8, 2015, from http://www.jstor.org/stable/3402067

Duda, J. (2013, January 11). Vote analysis shows why Flake–Carmona race was so close. *Arizona Capital Times.* Retrieved August 30, 2015, from http://azcapitoltimes.com/news/2013/01/11/jeff-flake-richard-carmona-vote-analysis-shows-why-it-was-so-close/

Faculty Sketch. (n.d.). Retrieved August 31, 2015, from Vanderbilt University School of Nursing: http://www.nursing.vanderbilt.edu/research/bios/buerhaus3.html

Ferguson, L. K. (2014). Susie Walking Bear Yellowtail: "Our Bright Morning Star" [Weblog]. Retrieved August 10, 2015, from http://montanawomenshistory.org/susie-walking-bear-yellowtail-our-bright-morning-star/

Fitzpatrick, M. A. (2015). The essence of nursing. *American Nurse Today supplement: The Essence of Nursing,* May 2015, 2–3.

Frank, M. (2002, March 31). The doctor is armed. *Time.* Retrieved August 30, 2015, from http://content.time.com/time/health/article/0,8599,221152,00.html

Frederick, S. (2014, May 14). Nursing in a new light. *TODAY Magazine.* Retrieved August 30, 2015, from http://today.mnsu.edu/2014/05/14/nursing-in-a-new-light/

From High School Dropout to Surgeon General—Thanks to BCC. (2002, October). *CUNY Matters.* Retrieved August 30, 2015, from http://www1.cuny.edu/portal_ur/news/cuny_matters/2002_october/carmona.html

Gelinas, L. (2015). Creating the environment for nursing excellence. *American Nurse Today supplement: The Essence of Nursing,* May 2015, 4–5.

Gennaro, S. (2014). Writing: Ensuring the stars align. *Journal of Nursing Scholarship, 46*(4), 217.

George, J. (2005). Madeleine Leininger. In J. George (Ed.), *Nursing theories: The base for professional nursing practice* (6th ed.; pp. 404–434). Old Tappan, NJ: Pearson Education.

Gross, L. (2013, July 10). More men join nursing field as social stigma disappears. *The Tennessean.* Retrieved August 30, 2015, from http://archive.tennessean. com/article/20130710/NEWS01/307100107/More-men-join-nursin g-field-social-stigma-disappears

Hall, H., & Manley, C. F. (2003, November 3). Buerhaus, Moses join Institute of Medicine. *Vanderbilt Register.* Retrieved August 30, 2015, from http://news. vanderbilt.edu/archived-news/register/articles/index-id=7485.html

Halloran, E. J. (2007). *Virginia Henderson.* Retrieved August 20, 2015, from http://www. aahn.org/gravesites/henderson.html

Harris, G. (2007, August 14). Ex-surgeon general's maverick side was bound to appear, friends say. *The New York Times.* Retrieved August 30, 2015, from http://www. nytimes.com/2007/08/14/washington/14carmona.html?_r=0

Hawkins, S., & Morse, J. (2014). The praxis of courage as a foundation for care. *Journal of Nursing Scholarship, 46*(4), 263–270.

Heavey, E. (2015). Differentiating statistical significance and clinical significance. *American Nurse Today, 10*(5), 26–28.

Hillestad, R., Bigelow, J., Bower, A., Girosi, F., Meill, R., Scoville, R., & Taylor, R. (2005). Can electronic medical record systems transform health care? Potential health benefits, savings, and costs. *Health Affairs, 24*(5), 1103–1117.

Hine, D. C. (1989). *Black women in white: Racial conflict and cooperation in the nursing profession 1890–1950.* Bloomington, IN: Indiana University Press.

Hine, D. C. (2004). Mabel Staupers. In S. Ware & S. Braukman (Eds.), *Notable American women* (pp. 611–612). Cambridge, MA: Belknap Press.

Houser, B. P., & Player, K. N. (2007). *Pivotal moments in nursing* (Vol. 2). Indianapolis, IN: Sigma Theta Tau International.

Hunter, R., & Carlson, E. (2014). Finding the fit: Patient-centered care. *Nursing Management, 45*(1), 38–43.

Institute of Medicine. (2011). *The future of nursing: Leading change, advancing health.* Washington, DC: National Academies Press.

Ives Erickson, J., Jones, D., & Ditomassi, M. (2013). Fostering nurse-led care. Indianapolis, IN: Sigma Theta Tau International.

Jennings, J. (2012, May 13). In celebration of national nursing week: The first women of healing. *Indian Country.* Retrieved August 10, 2015, from http:// indiancountrytodaymedianetwork.com/2012/05/13/celebration-nationa l-nursing-week-first-women-healing

Judd, D., Sitzman, K., & Davis, G. (2010). *A history of American nursing: Trends and eras.* Sudbury, MA: Jones and Bartlett Publishers.

Killen, T. (2013). It's all in the cards: Determining cultural preference information. *Nursing Management,* December 2013, 42–46.

Koch, H. B. (1951). *Militant angel.* New York, NY: Macmillan.

Lavinia Dock Collection. (n.d.). Retrieved July 3, 2015, from Alan Mason Chesney Medical Archives of The Johns Hopkins Medical Institutions: http://www. medicalarchives.jhmi.edu/papers/dock.html

Lee, C. (2007, July 11). Ex-surgeon general says White House hushed him. *The Washington Post.* Retrieved August 30, 2015, from http://www.washingtonpost. com/wp-dyn/content/article/2007/07/10/AR2007071001422.html

Lobo, M. (2005). Virginia Henderson. In J. George (Ed.), *Nursing theories: The base for professional nursing practice* (6th ed., pp. 87–112). Old Tappan, NJ: Pearson Education.

Marshall, H. E. (1972). *Mary Adelaide Nutting: Pioneer of modern nursing.* Baltimore, MD: Johns Hopkins University Press.

Mattson, J. E. (2005). Been there, done that. *Reflections on Nursing Leadership, 31*(1), 10–15.

McBride, A. B. (1996). In celebration of Virginia Avenuel Henderson. *Reflections in Nursing Leadership, 22*(1), 22–23.

McFarland, M. (2006). Madeleine Leininger. In A. M. Tomey & M. R. Alligood (Eds.), *Nursing theorists and their work* (6th ed.; pp. 472–496). St. Louis, MO: Mosby.

Medicare.gov. (2014). *Clinical process of care domain.* Retrieved August 30, 2015 from https://www.medicare.gov/hospitalcompare/data/clinical-process-of-care.html

MercyCollege. (2013). *Rev. Dr. Eugene Sawicki.* Available from https://legacyweb. mercy.edu/alumni-friends/60th-anniversary/

MercyCollege. (2010). *Alumni & Friends.* Retrieved August 30, 2015, from Mercy.edu: https://legacyweb.mercy.edu/alumni-friends/60th-anniversary/

Moffett, C. (2012). Nurses at the table: Bridging the gap from acute care to community. *Arizona Nurse, 65*(2), 1–12. Retrieved August 30, 2015, from http://nursingald. com/uploads/publication/pdf/15/AZ5_12.pdf

Montana Historical Society. (n.d.). *Susie Yellowtail.* Retrieved August 10, 2015, from http://mhs.mt.gov/Portals/11/education/Montanans/yellowtail2.pdf

Mosley, M. P. (2004). Estelle Massey Riddle Osborne. In S. Ware & S. Braukman (Eds.), *Notable American women* (pp. 491–493). Cambridge, MA: Belknap Press.

MSU News Service. (2014, November 11). MSU hires renowned nursing professor Peter Buerhaus. *Bozeman Daily Chronicle.* Retrieved August 30, 2015, from http:// www.bozemandailychronicle.com/news/montana_state_university/msu-hire s-renowned-nursing-professor-peter-buerhaus/article_b701bd6a-69f7-11e4-99ff- bb7ea80bf7cb.html

Murdock, G. (2006). Peter Buerhaus: Nursing workforce scholar. *NurseZone.* Retrieved August 30, 2015, from http://www.nursezone.com/printArticle. aspx?articleID=21602

Nelson, J., & Rosenthal, L. (2015). How nurses can help reduce hospital readmissions. *American Nurse Today supplement: The Essence of Nursing,* May 2015, 18–20.

Nightingale, F. (1992). *Notes on nursing: What it is and what it is not* (commemorative ed.). Philadelphia, PA: J.B. Lippincott Company.

Nightingale, F. (2012). *Florence Nightingale to her nurses* (facsimile reprint of 1914 ed.). Forgotten Books. Available from www.forgottenbooks.org

Nobody's Wife. (2006, October 5). Father Eugene Sawicki—The heart of Our Lady of Vilnius Parish [Weblog]. Retrieved August 30, 2015, from http://ausrosvartunyc. blogspot.com/2006/10/father-eugene-sawicki-heart-of-our.html

Nobody's Wife. (2007, August 25). A rare bird sighted at Robert Beddia's funeral [Weblog]. Retrieved August 30, 2015, from http://ausrosvartunyc.blogspot. com/2007/08/rare-bird-sighted-at-robert-beddias.html

Pima County Sheriff's Department. (2015). *Organization chart.* Retrieved August 30, 2015, from http://www.pimasheriff.org/files/8214/4293/7947/Complete_Org_Chart_large_092015.pdf

Palmer, J. (2011). Luther Christman: Legacy of a legend. *Reflections on Nursing Leadership, 37*(2). Retrieved August 22, 2015, from http://www.reflectionsonnursingleadership.org/Pages/Vol37_2_NoteFeat_Christman.aspx

Pear, R. (2002, March 27). Man in the news; A man of many professions—Richard Henry Carmona. *The New York Times.* Retrieved August 30, 2015, from http://www.nytimes.com/2002/03/27/us/man-in-the-news-a-man-of-many-pro fessions-richard-henry-carmona.html

Pederson, A.-E., & Garvey, M. (2002, July 8). Squaring off over nominee. *Los Angeles Times.* Available from http://pqasb.pqarchiver.com/latimes/results.html?st= advanced&QryTxt=&type=current&sortby=RELEVANCE&datetype=6&frommonth =07&fromday=08&fromyear=2002&tomonth=07&today=09&toyear=2002&By= &Title=squaring+off+over+nominee&at_curr=ALL&Sect=ALL

Pittman, E. (2005). *Luther Christman: A maverick nurse—A nursing legend.* Victoria, British Columbia: Trafford Publishing.

Porter-O'Grady, T. (2015). Through the looking glass: Predictive and adaptive capacity in a time of great change. *Nursing Management, 46*(6), 22–29.

Richards, L. (1911). *Reminiscences of Linda Richards, America's first trained nurse.* Boston, MA: Thomas Todd Company.

Robb, I. H. (1912). Nursing ethics: For hospital and private use (2nd ed.). Cleveland, OH: E. C. Koeckert.

Schorr, T., & Zimmerman, A. (1988). *Making choices: Taking chances.* St. Louis, MO: Mosby.

Scott, E. S. (2015). Leading change. In P. Yoder-Wise (Ed.), *Leading and managing in nursing* (6th ed.; pp. 305–319). St. Louis, MO: Mosby.

Selanders, L. (n.d.). Florence Nightingale: English nurse. Retrieved from http://www.britannica.com/biography/Florence-Nightingale

Shambaugh, R. (2012, April 23). Career advice: 5 ways to boost your political savvy and social intelligence. *Huffington Post.* Retrieved July 19, 2015, from http://www.huffingtonpost.com/rebecca-shambaugh/career-advice_b_1273688.html

Sherman, R. O. (2014). Dealing with difficult people. *American Nurse Today, 9*(5), 61–62.

Sherrod, D. (2015). Picking your priorities: An educational pathway. *Nursing Management,* February 2015, 12–14.

Smith, J., & Robinson, S. (2015). Beyond belief...redefining spirituality. *Nursing Management, 46*(2), 44–49.

Stasi, L. (1995, December 4). This man of cloth is bravest. *NY Daily News.* Retrieved August 30, 2015, from http://www.nydailynews.com/archives/news/man-clot h-bravest-article-1.692610

Stasi, L. (2007, March 5). Street preach. *The NY Post.* Retrieved September 4, 2015, from http://nypost.com/2007/03/05/street-preach/

Sullivan, E. (2002). In a woman's world. *Reflections on Nursing Leadership, 28*(3), 10–17.

Tomey, A., & Alligood, M. (2006). *Nursing theorists and their work* (6th ed.). St. Louis, MO: Mosby.

University of California, Department of Surgery. (2014). *Historical perspectives from the Department of Surgery.* San Francisco, CA: The Regents of the University of California. Retrieved August 30, 2015, from http://cohenlab.surgery.ucsf.edu/media/7369391/Loupes-Ceremony-2014-Booklet.pdf

Vanderbilt University, Department of Health Policy. (2015). *Peter I. Buerhaus, Ph.D.* Retrieved August 30, 2015, from https://medschool.vanderbilt.edu/health-policy/person/peter-i-buerhaus-phd

Voda, S. G. (2012). Remembering visionaries in nursing practice. *Nursing 2012, 42*(8), 1–3.

Volland, J. (2014). Creating a new healthcare landscape. *Nursing Management, 45*(4), 22–29.

Wacker Guido, G. (2015). Legal & ethical issues. In P. Yoder Wise (Ed.), *Leading & managing in nursing* (6th ed.; pp. 70–96). St. Louis, MO: Mosby.

Wesley, Y. (2015). Leadership competencies to reduce health disparities. *Nursing Management,* February 2015, 51–53.

Whitelaw, N. (1994). *Margaret Sanger: "Every Child a Wanted Child".* New York, NY: Dillon Press.

Whitman, W. (2015). *The Wound Dresser.* Retrieved September 6, 2015, from http://www.poetryfoundation.org/poem/237970

WhyIWantToBeANurse.org. (c. 2011). *Virginia Henderson.* Retrieved August 20, 2015, from http://www.whyiwanttobeanurse.org/nursing-theorists/virginia-henderson.php

Wilkie, K., & Moseley, E. (1969). *Frontier nurse: Mary Breckinridge.* New York, NY: Julian Messner

Williams, B. (1948). *Lillian Wald: Angel of Henry Street.* New York, NY: Julian Messner.

Wood, D. (2004). Surgeon General Richard Carmona began as RN. Retrieved August 30, 2015, from http://www.nursezone.com/search.aspx?q=richard%20carmona (link no longer active)

Yost, E. (1955). *American women of nursing* (rev. ed.). New York, NY: G. P. Putnam's Sons.

Index

Symbols

12 community essentials 116

A

advanced practice nursing 130, 165
advanced practice registered
    nurses (APRNs) 31, 36
Affordable Care Act
  Hospital Readmission Reduction
    Program 25
Agency for Healthcare Research
    and Quality (AHRQ) 155
American Academy of Medicine 73
American Academy of Nursing 130,
    132
American Anthropological
    Association 115
American Assembly for Men in
    Nursing 131

American Association of Critical-
    Care Nurses (AACN) 133
American Association of Nurse
    Midwives 58
American Birth Control League 71,
    73
American Board of Missions 3
American Committee for
    Devastated France
    (CARD) 51
American Indian Nurses
    Association 108
American Nurses Association
    (ANA) 34, 82, 91, 102, 127, 141
  discrimination 80–81, 91, 101, 131
  Hall of Fame 17, 108, 132
  House of Delegates 82, 91
  integration 17, 82, 91–92
  president of 40, 130
Apsáalooke 105, 106, 108
Armed Forces Nurse Corps 89
Army Nurse Corps 88–89, 127–128

Army School of Nursing 41, 119
assessment 106, 108–109, 165
Associated Alumnae of the United
States 45

B

Barton, Clara 7–11
and the American Red Cross 10
Civil War 8
delegation 12
disaster relief 12
paralells between Florence
Nightingale and 11
Bellevue Hospital 2, 19, 27, 39
Training School 33, 39, 43, 146
birth control 65–72
American Birth Control
League 71
Clinical Research Bureau 72, 73,
76
literature
Birth Control Review 70
Family Limitation 67–68
Woman and the New Race 70
methods
abortion 66
condom 65
diaphragm 72
pill 74
Board of Health 21, 56, 59
Booker T. Washington
Sanitarium 85
Boston City Hospital 2, 3, 4
School of Nursing 105
Breckinridge, Mary 49–58
Frontier Graduate School of
Midwifery 59
Frontier Nursing Service
(FNS) 55
Courier Service 56
influenza epidemic 50
Kentucky Committee for Mothers
and Children 54

political savvy 59–60
Brevan's Seven Change Factors 83
Bronx Community College
(BCC) 138
Buerhaus, Peter 153–156
contribution to professional
literature 155
economic accountability 156–157
Bureau of Indian Affairs
Hospital 106

C

Cadet Nurse Corps 81, 90–91, 111
Canyon Ranch Institute 141, 168
CARD (American Committee for
Devastated France) 51
caring and culture (transcultural
nursing) 115–116
Carmona, Richard 135–141
Canyon Ranch Institute 141
courage 140–141, 142–143
deputy sheriff 140–141
Ebola 141
Raoul & Lucy Carmona Memorial
Scholarship 139
surgeon general 139, 140–142
Carnegie Corporation 55, 58
Carnegie Foundation 29
Carnegie, Mary Elizabeth 95–102
contribution to professional
literature 103–104
American Journal of Nursing 101
*Disadvantaged Students in RN
Programs* 102
Nursing Outlook 102
*The Path We Tread: Blacks in
Nursing* 103
change agency 79, 82–83, 107, 165
Chi Eta Phi 17
Christman, Luther 125–132
Christman's Laws of Behavior 129
innovation 132–134
Rush Model 131

Christman's Laws of Behavior 129
civil rights 9
  academic integration 88
  military integration 81, 88–90
Civil War 8, 159
clinical nurse specialist (CNS) 112
Clinical Research Bureau 72, 73, 76
Clinical Scene Investigator (CSI)
        Academy 133
clinical significance 75
Code of Ethics for Nurses,
        Provisions 46–47
collaboration 5, 18, 121, 142, 166
College Settlement 21
Columbia University 40
  Teachers College 23, 29, 31, 34, 40,
        44, 52, 78, 97, 120, 146
computerized physician order
        entry (CPOE) 5
Comstock Laws 65, 74
conflict management 88, 90, 92–93,
        164
contribution to professional
        literature 35, 44, 103, 121–122,
        155, 165
Cooper Hospital School of
        Nursing 128
courage 140–141, 142–143, 164
Crimean War vii, 2, 88
cultural diversity 24–25, 165
cultural issues in nursing.
        See transcultural nursing

D

delegation 12–13, 164
disaster relief 11, 13, 51–52
discrimination
  gender 8, 126–127, 130, 132, 153
  racial 15, 77, 80, 87–90, 97–98, 99,
        100, 101, 106, 137
Dock, Lavinia 33–35
  contribution to professional
        literature 34, 35

Henry Street Settlement 34
  legislative advocacy 36
  social activism 34
Doyle, Mabel. *See* Keaton Staupers,
        Mabel
Duval Medical Center 99

E

Ebola 141
economic accountability 154,
        156–157, 165
education 21, 138, 155
  discrimination in, 88
  nursing 2, 5, 28, 29–31, 35, 37, 39,
        44, 81, 101, 130, 164
    Rush Model 131
  public health 25, 42, 71, 86, 140
  sex 67–68, 70, 73
  special 22
electronic medical records
        (EMRs) 4–5
emergency preparedness 12, 140,
        142
Emile, Ibrahim vii
ethics 46–47, 143, 148, 164

F

Florida A&M 98, 99, 100
Florida Association of Colored
        Graduate Nurses
        (FACGN) 101
Florida State Nurses Association
        (FSNA) 101
Franklin County Public
        Hospital 106
Freedman's Hospital 78, 85, 97
Frontier Graduate School of
        Midwifery 59
Frontier Nursing Service (FNS) 52,
        55, 58–59, 60
  Courier Service 51, 56

G

Goodrich, Annie 37–41
 army hospitals 41–42
 health promotion 42–43
 Henry Street Settlement 40
 Yale Graduate School of
   Nursing 41
Grand Duchess Louise 9
Griswold vs. Connecticut 74

H

Hampton Robb, Isabel 43–46
 contributions to professional
   literature 44
 nursing ethics 46–47
Hampton University 98
Harlem Hospital Nursing
   School 78
Harvard 37
 Liberal Club 73
 School of Public Health 155
health promotion 22, 42–43, 165
Henderson, Virginia 119–122
 contribution to professional
   literature 121, 122
 Henry Street Settlement 120
 nursing need theory 121
 patient-centered care 123
Henry Street Settlement 20, 22, 23,
   25, 34, 40, 120
Higgins, Maggie Louisa. See Sanger,
   Margaret
Highland and Islands Medical
   Service 53
*History of American Red Cross
   Nursing* 35
History of Nursing 35
Homer G. Phillips Hospital 77, 78
Hospital Consumer Assessment of
   Healthcare Providers and
   Systems (HCAHPS) 123, 157
hospital design 39

Hospital Economics 29, 30, 40, 44
Hospital for Women and
   Children 2, 15
Howard University 78, 85, 97, 102

I

Illinois Training School for
   Nurses 44
innovation 132–134, 165
Institute for Social Research 129
Institute of Medicine (IOM) 5, 31,
   36
International Convention of
   Geneva. See Red Cross
International Council of Nurses 34,
   101

J

Japan 3, 6, 72
Jefferson Hospital 86
Johns Hopkins University 29, 155
 Training School for Nurses 28,
   33, 44

K

Keaton Staupers, Mabel 85–91
 conflict management 92–93
 personality types 92–93
Kentucky Committee for Mothers
   and Children 54
King's College Hospital 3
Kotter's 8-Step Model 83

L

Lancaster, Mary Elizabeth.
   See Carnegie, Mary Elizabeth
leadership in nursing. See
   also nurse leader
   implications; nursing,
   leadership competencies

Nightingale's legacy 163
Nightingale's legacy to vii
legislative advocacy 36, 107, 165
Leininger, Madeleine 111–115
  qualitative research 114
  transcultural nursing 113–114,
    115–116
levels of personality 148
Lincoln School 78, 96
Lower East Side 21, 23, 25, 34

M

Mahoney, Mary Eliza 15–17
  quality patient care 17
managed care 24–25, 58
Manhattan College 146
Manhattan Eye and Ear
    Hospital 64
Mary Eliza Mahoney Family Life
    Center 17
Massachusetts General Hospital
    (MGH) 2
  Professional Practice
      Environment model 6
Massey Riddle Osborne, Estelle 77–
    82
  ANA Board of Directors 82
  change agency 82–83
    Brevan's Seven Change
        Factors 83
    Kotter's 8-Step Model 83
  National Nursing Council for War
      Service 81
Mead, Margaret 112
Medicare 25, 123, 157
Mercy College 145, 149
Methodist Hospital School of
    Nursing 126
Metropolitan Life Insurance
    Company 25, 58–59
midwives 51, 53, 59, 67, 97
Military Nurse Corps 128
Minnesota State Mankato 153

Minority Program Advisory
    Committee 102
Mount St. Scholastica College 112
Mudget Hospital 85

N

National Association of Colored
    Graduate Nurses
    (NACGN) 16, 79–80, 86, 92,
    96
  Mary Eliza Mahoney Award 17,
    82–83
National News 87
National Birth Control League 67,
    71
National Council of Negro
    Women 80
National Disaster Medical
    System 141
National First Aid Association 11
National Health Care Workforce
    Commission 155
National League for Nursing
    Education. *See* National
    League for Nursing (NLN)
National League for Nursing
    (NLN) 31, 81, 82, 100, 102,
    129, 131
National Nurse Response 141
National Nursing Council for War
    Service 81
National Organization for
    Public Health Nursing
    (NOPHN) 88
Navy Nurse Corps 88, 90, 97
New York City Fire Department
    (FDNY) 146
New York Hospital Training
    School 19, 38, 39
New York Infirmary, Women's
    Medical College 20
New York Juvenile Asylum 20
New York Medical Society 73

New York Postgraduate Hospital 38
New York State Guard 147
New York Woman's Hospital 44
Nightingale, Florence
  assessment 106
  change agency 79, 82
  and Clara Barton 9-10, 11
  conflict management 92-93
  contribution to professional
      literature 103, 122, 155
  courage 143
  health promotion 22
  innovation 132, 134
  legislative advocacy 36
  and Linda Richards 2
  and Mary Adelaide Nutting 30
  Notes on Nursing 27, 46, 103
  political savvy 59-60
  quality patient care 16, 17
  spirituality 150
Nightingale Fund 2
Norfolk Protestant Hospital 120
Northwest Health Foundation 133
nurse case managers 25
nurse leader implications
  assessment's importance
      (Yellowtail) 108-110
    leadership competency and 165
  care delivery excellence
      (Mahoney) 17-18
    leadership competency and 166
  caring and culture
      (Leininger) 115-116
    leadership competency and 164
  change agent (Osborne) 82-84
    leadership competency and 165
  collegiate education promotion
      (Nutting) 31-32
    leadership competency and 164
  courage (Carmona) 142-144
    leadership competency and 164
  cultural diversity (Wald) 24
    leadership competency and 164

  dealing with difficult people
      (Staupers) 92-94
  delegation's importance
      (Barton) 12
    leadership competency and 164
  disaster relief advocacy
      (Barton) 12-13
  economic accountability
      (Buerhaus) 156-158
    leadership competency and 165
  ethical behavior (Robb) 46-47
    leadership competency and 164
  global collaboration
      (Richards) 5-6
    leadership competency and 166
  health promotion (Goodrich) 42
    leadership competency and 165
  innovation (Christman) 132-134
    leadership competency and 165
  legislative advocacy (Dock) 36
    leadership competency and 165
  managed care leverage
      (Wald) 24-25
  patient-centered care
      (Henderson) 123-124
    leadership competency and 164
  political savvy (Breckinridge) 59-
      61
    leadership competency and 164
  professional literature
      contributions
      (Carnegie) 103-104
    leadership competency and 165
  recordkeeping system for patients
      (Richards) 4-5
  spirituality (Sawicki) 150-151
    leadership competency and 164
  statistical analysis (Sanger) 75-76
    leadership competency and 165
nurse-midwives 52-53, 54, 56,
    58-59
nurse-patient relationships 121, 124
Nurses' Associated Alumnae 34

Nurses Directory 16
nurse-sensitive indicators 75, 134,
    155, 157
nursing
  collaboration 5, 18, 142, 166
  education 2, 5, 28, 29, 30–32, 35,
      37, 39, 41, 44, 99–100, 164
  Rush Model 131
  ethics 46–47, 143, 148, 164
  leadership competencies
  assessment 106, 108–109, 165
  change agency 79, 82–83, 107,
      165
  collaboration 121
  conflict management 88, 90,
      92–93, 164
  contribution to professional
      literature 35, 44, 103, 121–122,
      155, 165
  courage 140–141, 142–143, 164
  cultural diversity 24–25, 165
  delegation 12, 164
  disaster relief 11, 13, 51–52
  economic accountability 154,
      156–157, 165
  education. *See* nursing,
      education
  global collaboration.
      See nursing, collaboration
  health promotion 42–43, 165
  innovation 132–134, 165
  legislative advocacy 36, 107, 165
  political savvy 59–60, 89–90, 164
  quality patient care 17–18, 166
  recordkeeping 4–5, 22, 55, 58, 72
  spirituality 106–107, 108, 146,
      148–150, 164
  statistical analysis 54–55, 57, 72,
      75–76, 165
  transcultural nursing 113,
      115–116, 164

Transcultural Nursing
    Society 115
men in. *See* Christman, Luther;
    See Sawicki, Eugene;
    See Carmona, Richard;
    See Buerhaus, Peter
in the military 8, 11, 41–42, 89, 119,
    127–128, 137–138
need theory 121
research 114, 121–122
Nutting, Mary Adelaide 27–31
  American Journal of Nursing 29
  and Florence Nightingale 30
  nursing education 29, 30, 31–32

O

The Ohio State University College
    of Nursing 141

P

Partners Investing in Nursing's
    Future grant 133
Patent Office 8–9
patient-centered care 120, 123, 164
Pennsylvania Hospital School of
    Nursing for Men 126
Pennsylvania School for Health
    and Social Work 86
personality types 92–93
Planned Parenthood 74
political savvy 59–60, 89–90, 164
practitioner-teacher 128, 130
professional literature
    contributions.
      See contributions to
      professional literature
public health
  Community Health Project 17
  Community Health
      Representatives Outreach
      Program 107
public health nurses 22, 52, 56

Q

quality patient care 17–18, 123, 164, 166

R

recordkeeping 4–5, 22, 55, 58, 72
Red Cross 9
  American 10, 12, 35, 50, 57, 89
Richards, Linda 1–5
  and Florence Nightingale 2
  global collaboration 5
  Japan 3
  recordkeeping 4
Robert Wood Johnson
      Foundation 133
Rockefeller Foundation 86, 98, 99
Rosenwald Fellowship 78
Rosenwald Foundation 78
Royal Infirmary of Edinburgh 3
Rush University 131, 168
  Rush Model 131

S

Sanger, Margaret 63–72
  birth control 65–72
    American Birth Control
        League 71
    Brownsville Clinic 68
    literature
      Birth Control Review 70
      Family Limitation 67–68
      Woman and the New Race 70
    methods
      abortion 66
      condoms 65
      diaphragms 72
      pill 74
    Clinical Research Bureau 72, 73, 76
    and H. G. Wells 70
    and J. Noah Slee 71

Japan 72
    Planned Parenthood 74
    statistical analysis 72, 75–76
Sawicki, Eugene 145–149
  levels of personality 148
  New York City Fire Department
      (FDNY) 146, 148
  Our Lady of Vilnius 147, 149
  September 11, 2001 148
  spirituality 146, 148–150
    seven Cs 150
school nurses 22
segregation 80, 96, 100
  in the military 89–90
September 11, 2001 140, 148
A Short History of Nursing 35
Sigma Theta Tau 122, 143, 148
Sloane Maternity Hospital 38
social intelligence 60–61
Socialist 63, 66, 71
Social Reform Club 23
Society of Superintendents of
      Training Schools 34, 45
Southern Regional Education
      Board 130
spirituality 106–107, 108, 146, 148–
      150, 164
Standards of Practice 42, 109
Standards of Professional Nursing
      Practice 13
Standards of Professional
      Performance 13
St. Anthony's School of Nursing 111
statistical analysis 54–55, 57, 58, 72,
      75–76, 165
  certainty level 75
  Clinical Research Bureau 72, 73,
      76
  clinical significance 75
  probability value 75
  statistical significance 75
  type I error 76
  type II error 76
statistical significance 75

St. Augustine 150
St. George's Episcopal Church 71
St. Joseph's Hospital 112
St. Louis Municipal Visiting
  Nurses 78
St. Luke's Hospital 39, 50, 56
St. Paul's House 44
St. Philip Hospital 97, 100
St. Thomas' Hospital 2
surgeon general
  of the army 88–89, 90–91, 94,
    127–128
  Carmona, Richard 139, 140–142
Sutliffe, Irene 19
Syracuse University 98

T

Temple University 128
Textbook of Nursing 28
The Joint Commission (TJC) 123
transcultural nursing 113, 115–116,
  164
  community essentials 116
Transcultural Nursing Society 115
Tuberculosis and Health
  Association 86
type I error 76
type II error 76

U

University of California at San
  Francisco (UCSF) 139
University of Cincinnati 112–113
University of Colorado 113
University of Iowa 155

University of Michigan 129, 154
University of Pennsylvania 142, 168
University of Toronto 98
University of Washington 113

V

value-based purchasing 123,
  157–158
Vanderbilt University 130
Veterans Administration 97

W

Wald, Lillian 19–24
  and Albert Einstein 23
  cultural diversity 24–25
  Henry Street Settlement 22
  managed care 24–25
Walking Bear Yellowtail, Susie 105–
  109
  assessment 108–109
  Award for Outstanding Nursing
    Health Care 107
  spirituality 106–107
Wayne State University 114, 154
West Virginia State College 97
Whitman, Walt 159–161
Woodstock College 146
World War I 70, 119
World War II 88, 127
"The Wound Dresser" 160–162

Y

Yale Graduate School of Nursing 41
Yankton State Hospital 128